Peak Experie

the Road Le:

MW01120107

Unexpected

ALLEN MASTERS

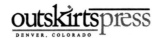

DENVER, COLORADO

Outskirts Press, Inc.
http://www.outskirtspress.com

Paperback ISBN: 978-1-4787-1198-8
Hardcover ISBN: 978-1-4327-9895-6

Outskirts Press and the "OP" logo are trademarks belonging to Outskirts Press, Inc.

PRINTED IN THE UNITED STATES OF AMERICA

Contents

Acknowledgments

The idea for this book came from my 15-year younger half-brother, Tony, who urged me to put my life experiences in writing so that he could "get to know me better." Although he never mentioned why this was important to him, I suspect it had a lot to do with our mother, by then deceased, who had a pronounced tendency to describe my journey through life in unrealistically glowing terms. Here is the way I experienced it, in memoir (episodic) rather than autobiographical (timeline) form.

In keeping with the fact that much of my life was dominated by my medical career, the content of this volume has been reviewed—or contributed to—by several of my professional colleagues, especially Doctors Robert Sherins, Alain Traig, and Vernon Weldon. The greatest influence in my professional life was wielded by the Professor, who has his own chapter herein.

Grateful acknowledgment is made of permission by Random House Publishers to cite passages from Michael Crichton's novel, *Disclosure*.

Preface

The year 1937 in America was noteworthy for being the time of the second sharp downturn in the Great Depression. It was also the time when I was born. The place was Glendale, a suburban village north of Cincinnati in conservative southwestern Ohio. My father's family had lived there since 1855, when the village was founded. My family was upper-middle class; my paternal grandfather and his father and brother were Harvard graduates and patent lawyers. My maternal grandfather was a family doctor. With such a background it seemed the natural thing for me to do was to marry the equivalent of the girl next door, practice one of the professions, and raise our three wonderful children in a century-old, large frame house on a quarter-acre lot in Glendale.

It didn't happen; not even close.

Both sets of grandparents were divorced several years before I was born. This was a period when "nice people" (as my mother would say) did not do that. Both my maternal grandmother and her only son, my uncle, died of mysterious causes about the time I was born. My mother was 20 when she had me, her firstborn. She was a Wellesley dropout who expected to be a happily married housewife and mother. My father attended three different colleges before entering medical school in Cincinnati. He sired me and my two-and-a-half-year younger brother before getting divorced from my mother and heading for the West Coast, never to return to live.

The alimony, child support, and what little my mother was able to earn did not begin to support an upper-middle-class existence in Glendale, where my brother and I were raised. We were the poor relatives. I was too embarrassed to invite my school friends over to play or for dinner; I had no compunction about visiting their houses. Most of my clothes were hand-me-downs. When my social peers went to dancing school and to summer camp as a matter of course, I had a brief stint at each but did not continue due to lack of money. I like to say that I was raised in genteel poverty. We never went hungry or were evicted because we could not pay the rent, but it was close.

After six years at the Glendale elementary school, my mother attempted to improve my lot by enrolling me in Walnut Hills High, Cincinnati's public college preparatory school. Transportation was difficult; I did exceptionally poorly in the obligatory Latin; and early adolescence was a torment. Relief came when my stepfather of two years got a job transfer to Europe and I was parked, at age 15, at Saint Peter's, a private school in New York State. At the end of my initial semester there, the English master wrote in my yearbook: "Rags to riches in three months. Wow!" It was true. I had found my niche.

As the following pages will tell, my subsequent life has been filled with unexpected twists and turns, some nearly fatal. The adventurer in me has been more than satisfied. And I have become wealthy, not so much monetarily as in the experiences I have had. Glendale was a starting point, not a destination or way of life. My three-quarter-century existence has encompassed things so far removed from there that I feel as though I have lived several lifetimes in the course of one lifespan.

This is a memoir of those experiences in the form of first-person essays. The essays are grouped by subject matter, but can be read in any order because each is a standalone.

Why I Hated Princeton

We live in an age when some of America's most success-ful people—Bill Gates of Microsoft and Apple founder Steve Jobs come to mind—are college dropouts. Nevertheless, the mainstream media's constant drumbeat is about getting into college. They say that a number of parents will do anything short of murder to get their kid into an Ivy League school. Perhaps some do commit felonies for the sake of this goal but are understandably reluctant to crow about it.

In the face of this, it may seem that I'm going directly against the grain by downplaying and even denying the as-sumed virtues of one of the leading Ivy League schools, Princeton University. Is this simple gratuitous iconoclasm or is there more to it?

In 1955 I was a high school senior at a small Episcopalian private school in Peekskill, New York. Most of the students, myself included, were on scholarship. Money was scarce. Because I had done well after transferring in as a sophomore, my faculty advisors told me to shoot for the top. I did. I ap-plied to Harvard, Yale, Princeton, and Stanford. I was accepted at all four, the only sour note being an alternate acceptance at Harvard. The choice was easy: Princeton gave me a full-tuition scholarship and a job; the others less or nothing in the way of financial assistance.

Because of constraints on money and time, I hadn't visited any of the four campuses. I had no on-the-ground appreciation for what I was getting myself into. But I did envision a positive experience. I felt extremely fortunate.

Negative feelings commenced almost as soon as my foot hit campus. It wasn't due to a particular thing or two; it was more like a bad fit from multiple perspectives. Was my failure to thrive mainly due to my own shortcomings or was there more to the story, such as Princeton not always deserving its sterling reputation?

By failure to thrive I don't mean it in an outward sense. I got satisfactory grades, had friends as roommates, and was a member of Tiger Inn, one of the top five eating clubs. But there was something missing, something large, something which, for lack of a better term, could be described as existential. What passed for success in the eyes of others was to me unfulfilling, meaningless, or offensive. That I was not alone in having such feelings is suggested by the number of dropouts in the freshman and sophomore years.

It has been more than a half century since my Princeton days, yet I still have these feelings despite assurances from others that they would pass. I felt cheated when roommates from medical training would talk glowingly about their college experiences and rate them well above those of medical school. I felt just the opposite. Was it the college or was it me and those who dropped out?

There must have been at least a thousand reasons why I hated Princeton, but recounting a handful of the top offenders will give the flavor of my emotions about that place. It may also provide hints as to why the fit was so unsatisfactory.

Things got off to a bad start almost immediately. It was D-Day, H-Hour, when, suitcase in hand, I located my freshman dormitory. It was a turn-of-the-century attempt to create a four-story, square-shaped, courtyard-containing Roman building of red brick. It housed the poor: freshman scholarship students like myself. As I climbed the three flights of creaky wooden stairs to the top, I noticed how utterly uncharming the building was. I entered a corner room with bedrooms at either end. Two of my roommates were there; they shared one of the bedrooms, which had been designed for one person, not two. It was cramped living. My two roommates gave each other a knowing look as they nodded towards the door to the other bedroom. As the last to arrive, I got to share this other bedroom.

I was stupefied as I entered. The other occupant had arranged his bed, bureau, and night table such that they occupied nearly three-fourths of the small room. The accoutrements, such as the bedside lamp base in the shape of a cartoon piggy, suggested that his socialization hadn't progressed much beyond the second grade. I was becoming more incensed by the moment. Then in he walked.

Slight, bespectacled, with the look of a loner about him, he asked why I was moving his furniture around. I replied that it should be glaringly apparent why I was doing it and that I would appreciate his help. He behaved as though his wants should unquestionably come first. His speech was marred by a pronounced stammer, something that would ordinarily evoke empathy but in his case became an object of ridicule. He roomed alone during the sophomore year before dropping out.

Ever since collecting stamps as a boy, I had noticed the faces on the US presidential series. I had been struck by a countenance other than Washington, Lincoln, and the Roosevelts; it was that of Woodrow Wilson, elected US president in 1912 after having been president of Princeton from 1902 to 1910. Unlike the aforementioned, who displayed a mien of authority and credibility, Wilson managed to look pious and pompous simultaneously. He appeared every bit the Presbyterian do-gooder he was, an unswerving idealist in foreign affairs when a large dose of pragmatism is the only thing that matters most of the time. His stern visage looked down at you all over the campus; it was like a pre-Orwellian Big Brother was watching. I developed an aversion to all that he stood for.

One of those aversions was the much-touted seminar system that he instituted. Groups of six or eight students and a faculty preceptor would meet weekly to discuss the course material. The seminars always felt contrived and artificial to me. In practice, they were an open invitation for overly talkative suck-butts to BS their way through the class. Never once did I get the sense that understanding and knowledge were advanced by the system.

There were powerful reasons why I stuck it out at Princeton. My upbringing and the sense of society at that time led to the belief that a college degree was all-important to future success. If you didn't get a college diploma, you were likely to fall off the edge of the earth and never be seen again. Or so it seemed.

One of my Princeton-induced wounds was largely

self-inflicted. During my sophomore year it came time to choose a major field of study for junior and senior years. I had learned early on that geography was out because it was considered insufficiently academic for the ivied halls of Princeton. (UCLA professor of geography, Jared Diamond, author of *Guns, Germs, and Steel* and other bestsellers, would not have found a home there.) So I asked myself what I would most like to do to while away the hours, days, weeks, and months till I could walk out with a sheepskin. I chose English based on the fact that I liked to read novels and that, surely, they would constitute much of the discipline as it was understood in academia. I was wrong. The short-lived pleasures of wishful thinking precluded my doing even a cursory search into the requirements for majoring in English. Had I looked, I would have found that modern novels took a backseat to such hedonistic pleasures as Beowulf in Old English, reams of poetry from the preceding five centuries, and plays that could really be understood only by insiders to the court of England's King James in the 17th century. Chaucer's *Canterbury Tales* in Middle English—"Whan that Aprille with his shoures soote..."—did get a little racy from time to time when characters were swyving one another, but on the whole it didn't seem worth the slog. The crowning blow came when it was time to read—and comprehend—the later novels of James Joyce. Some of my classmates swooned over such passages as "A yellow dressinggown, ungirdled, was sustained gently behind him on the midmorning air. He held the bowl aloft and intoned: *Introibo ad altere Dei...*" in the novel *Ulysses* and claimed to be enraptured by "Countlessness of livestories have nether fallen by this page, flick as flowflakes, letters from aloft, like a waast wizard all of whirlworlds..." in *Finnegan's Wake*.

At the end of two years of such torture, the Princeton English department and I agreed that I was not among the literati despite their best ministrations. I wrote my senior thesis on the social novels of the 1930s. John Steinbeck's books come to mind. This was like taking a poke at the eye of the faculty. They were much more interested in the esoterica of previous centuries and in the purported symbolism in Ernest Hemingway's novels. I am thankful that they took pity on me and gave me a gentlemanly C so I could walk out the door a free man. I left a mailing address so that my diploma could be forwarded and left two weeks before the graduation ceremonies. I never returned.

On rare occasions, perhaps once every five years, I revisit Princeton in my mind's eye. I visualize the constant reminders of Woodrow Wilson, all as irritating as the screech of fingernails on a blackboard. Every time I returned after a semester or summer break, I felt like the protagonist in a bleak, sepia-toned black-and-white movie showing a convict returning to prison. I have the sense of walking from one building to another on campus, noting how little of what I see has the least appeal to me.

In my life after Princeton, nothing seemed to connect the two. Nobody in medical school, surgical training, my career in the Army, or my post-Army job as a city-county health director seemed to know or care that I had a diploma from Princeton. All they were interested in was whether I had a college degree. Period. To be a college graduate was a bureaucratic requirement, nothing more.

The year 2000 brought two revelations that had strong resonance in me. The first was the vacuousness of the millennial doomsday predictions. The second was the NPR broadcast I happened to hear as I was parking my car in a Costco parking lot. Instead of going into the store right away, I sat spellbound for 45 minutes as I listened to a recorded speech given to the Commonwealth Club of California. It was given by a Doctor (in education) Marty Nemko on the subject of higher education.

Marty, as I'll call him, came across as a streetwise verbal pugilist who disarms his opponents (or audiences) with self-deprecating humor delivered with a New York accent. He announced at the outset that he was going to question the educational assumptions that his audience of highly educated elites held as inviolable. And he did. Repeatedly. He turned the usual arguments about the value of a college education on their head. He also accused colleges and universities, as a group, of not practicing truth in advertising. In fact, as Marty indicated, the claims were so specious that, if trotted before a regulatory body as an ordinary business might be, they would be adjudged in violation of the law.

Finally, in some 40 years after graduation from Princeton, I felt vindicated. There was a kindred spirit on the planet. He had impeccable credentials to make his claims. And he was not afraid to challenge the conventional wisdom. The audience gave him tepid applause. But I, for one, would give him highest marks. As Marty said, institutions of higher learning are fundamentally businesses, and should be regarded as such. Stripped of the myths and examined in the cold light of day, Princeton and its esteemed rivals would appear unworthy of the adulation now heaped upon them.

These are a few of the many reasons that I hated Princeton. As always, *caveat emptor*.

Beneath the White Coat

Q. What do you call the student who finishes medical school dead last in the graduating class?

A. Doctor.

A newspaper columnist notices that the office nurse says: "Doctor will see you now." He wonders why she does not say "The doctor will see you now" or "Dr. Jones will see you now." She just says "Doctor." Finally he gets it. After all, one does not say "the Jesus."

A real estate agent was driving me around town to look at homes for sale. After spending a fruitless morning, we went out again in the afternoon. Nothing seemed appropriate for me. The explanation came with her question: "Doctor, how many children did you say you had?" I had told her in the morning that I had no children and no spouse. All she heard was the word "Doctor"; she then filled in the blanks. The home tour ended shortly thereafter.

The confusion of image with reality is pervasive. Think of the occasional news reports of charlatans successfully posing as MDs for years before it is revealed that they have not spent a day in medical school. But they have an ingratiating bedside manner.

Or think back to the days of the immensely popular *Marcus Welby, MD* TV show. Thousands of viewers contacted the network seeking medical advice from Dr. Welby, who, in their opinion, was the best doctor in the land. Their would-be doctor was an actor, no more.

The reality, of course, often differs from the image, sometimes strikingly so. It is a decidedly mixed bag. The following vignettes provide revealing glimpses beneath the white coat.

PSYCHIATRY IN MEDICAL SCHOOL

I started medical school in 1959 at the University of California San Francisco, better known as UCSF. I didn't know what specialty I might eventually choose, but I was sure that it would not be psychiatry, among others. This was not due to any particular event, but to sensing that it wouldn't suit my personality. My premonition would be tested in the next four years of school.

On the first day of school, we freshmen students sat in a lecture hall where we were presented with such things as a formal welcome from the provost, an aristocratic Scottish anatomist of the old school, and a movie of an abdominal operation, during which a future roommate fainted when droplets of blood popped out from the long incision into the skin. All but one of the presentations were in the same vein: welcomes to the serious professional world we were now entering.

The exception was in the form of a revelation of what we were like as a typical medical school class, which was made by an assistant professor of psychiatry. Dr. Fiberboard told us, in so many words, that we were socially underdeveloped as a consequence of concentrating on our studies as premed students rather than enjoying college life as a normal student would. In other words, don't get smug about the glowing descriptions of your potential as future doctors as presented by the other welcomers. That we all have weaknesses, including the faculty of a leading medical school, was revealed several months later when the *San Francisco Chronicle* ran a front-page story about a UCSF psychiatry professor caught peeping into the men's toilet stalls in nearby Golden Gate Park. We never saw or heard of Dr. Fiberboard again.

Unlike all the other clinical specialties, psychiatry was taught—both by lecture and by individual encounters with patients—in all four years of medical school. The other clinical specialties were reserved for our junior and senior years. I don't recall a rationale being given for this. By implication, psychiatry was either more important, more difficult to teach, or both.

I had expected that, with so much emphasis on psychiatry, we would have been given a thorough grounding in the basics. We weren't. Instead, we were given abstruse lectures on things unrelated to the basics of clinical medicine and told to buy Silvano Arieti's multi-author text on psychiatry. The latter showed not only the unevenness of the multi-author approach but also the fragmented state of psychiatry, with its many "schools."

As a sophomore, I was assigned to spend weekly hour-long sessions with a 13-year-old girl—an outpatient psychiatric patient. No guidance was offered on what I was supposed to do as the doctor. I asked the patient why she was at the clinic. She said that she was told to come there. She was vague and uncommunicative. She appeared to be passive, downcast, and sullenly resentful that she was made to come to the clinic. When I conveyed this to a faculty member after the session with the patient and asked what my role should be—i.e., What should I do?—I was told: "Talk to her." "About what?" "Just talk." "There doesn't appear to be anything that either one of us wants to talk about." "Just talk." Subsequent sessions were spent mainly in silence after several fruitless attempts to begin a dialogue.

In the third year of school, the first clinical year after two years of basic sciences, we students went to the county hospital, San Francisco General. As well as brief stints in medicine, surgery, and other specialties such as obstetrics, we spent several weeks in psychiatry on the inpatient ward, where we worked up three patients each and met with a faculty member who demonstrated his approach to a particular patient. The only useful thing I got from this was how to recognize hesitation marks on the wrist. The case in point was a young woman who allegedly tried to slit her wrist in a suicide attempt, but whose wrist bore several superficial cuts intended to attract attention to her plight, which was, as I recall, problems with her husband or boyfriend.

At the end of the academic quarter, our grades were posted. In addition to the usual A's, B's, C's, and occasional D's was an F, conspicuous because it was so unusual a grade. It was mine. I was totally taken aback. It would not have surprised me if it was a C or even a D, but an F? Hadn't I attended all the sessions with the faculty members, done the patient workups and whatever else was required? Had there been any warnings that my work was not up to par?

I scheduled an appointment to discuss the situation with the county hospital's chief of psychiatry, Dr. Mistri. Dr. Mistri, who seemed to be in his early forties, had what could be described as a seemingly honest face, with a forehead that could be deeply furrowed to express concern. I explained why I had asked to see him, which was what had caused me to fail the course and what I could do about it, especially when I was facing the imminent prospect of applying for an internship.

Dr. Mistri appeared to be unprepared to answer such a basic question. He tried to evade answering it. I persisted, full well knowing that, in that era, a medical student was virtually powerless in front of a faculty member. I pointed out that I had no inkling that my performance was so below par that I was given a failing grade. As he himself said, I was the first student in 500 to get a failing grade. He looked through some files, then gave me three reasons, which I demolished, one by one. One reason, according to him, was that my workup reports were "probably" unsatisfactory, that they "probably" were not adequately expressed. I replied that I was an English major at Princeton and therefore could probably express myself as well as a biology major from UC Berkeley. He then moved on to other reasons, or excuses, which were similarly dealt with.

What explains such behavior from a presumably acceptable faculty member? I don't know for sure, but I have an idea. I did pretty much the same things as my classmates, yet only I got a failing grade. But I had done something in addition—I spoke often and loudly to my classmates about how little esteem I had for psychiatry, at least as I had seen it at UCSF. I undoubtedly had been overheard by others, such as psychiatry residents and faculty members, who may have passed the word on to Dr. Mistri.

There is another possible dynamic: I have not got a poker face, and my body language gives me away, even when I try to control it. I learned as a freshman medical student that I could not win even at petty penny-ante poker: The other players could read my hand by reading my face. Perhaps the sessions with the various clinical faculty members gave me away: They may have seen all too clearly how little I respected their specialty.

The upshot of all this was that I was allowed to work up another three patients during the Christmas vacation. Unsurprisingly, I then received a passing grade, even though the workup reports were virtually identical to those I had written previously. Power ruled. The irony, of course, is that psychiatrists, as a rule, consider themselves politically liberal, yet this one apparently went to considerable lengths to stifle freedom of expression and peaceful dissent.

As a senior medical student, it was still unclear to me what I was supposed to do with the patients to whom I was assigned. Intuitively, I clung to the model of clinical medicine, a model that was relevant regardless of specialty: diagnosis, prognosis, and treatment, in that order. So I asked a faculty member how to go about making a psychiatric diagnosis. Instead of helping me make a diagnosis, he rebuked me for even posing the question. He intimated that it was wrong, virtually unethical, to "pin" a diagnosis on a patient because that would create the potential for saddling the patient with a mistaken categorization. I thought: Wasn't this a perfect way to flounder around endlessly, to avoid accountability?

It was not by accident that I chose future medical training in such a way as to have as little to do with psychiatry as possible.

TENNIS GAME

She was an attractive upper-middle-class wife and mother of two small children who lived in one of the tony suburbs of the East Bay of San Francisco. She began having strange symptoms involving her face. Her doctor referred her to a neurologist who, after some x-rays, diagnosed a benign tumor on her brain that was pressing on several cranial nerves and causing her symptoms. To let the tumor grow larger would probably lead to permanent damage to the nerves. To preclude this from happening, it was necessary to surgically remove the tumor, a tricky operation because of its location on the brain stem.

In 1963 I was a surgical intern at the University of California San Francisco Medical Center. I spent a month's rotation on neurosurgery, during which time the woman became one of my patients. She had been referred to the medical center as the patient of one of the leading professors, presumably to get the best care available in Northern California. The neurosurgery resident and I would assist the professor in the care of this patient.

As part of my duties, I was required to prepare her for surgery by shaving her nicely coiffed blond hair, which was one of her most attractive features. But of course it would eventually regrow and hide the surgical scar. She would regain her beauty.

At eight the next morning, the operation began. The surgeon—the professor—told the resident and me that he expected to complete the operation by noon. This was of concern because he had an important engagement elsewhere in the early afternoon.

To get to the site of the tumor, the surgeon cut into the right rear of the neck. Most of the bleeding was controlled by pressure or electric cauterization. However, there was one persistent bleeder that was resistant to control by the usual methods. It was necessary to stanch the bleeding before proceeding. The bleeder was particularly recalcitrant. The surgeon was unexpectedly forced to spend a great deal of time isolating and finally tying off the bleeder. He kept his eye on the clock.

Finally the area of the tumor came into view. It was an off-white sphere about the size of a hazelnut protruding back from the center of the brain stem, the narrow part of the brain that connects to the spinal cord. Despite the depths of the affected area, it was possible to get a clear view of the cranial nerves coming off each side of the brain stem. They looked like narrow pieces of twine hanging on either side of the tumor. The ones that were revealed controlled the eye muscles and the muscles of the face.

It was not possible to cut the tumor off at the base and pull it out. Trying to do so would risk injuring the brain stem and pushing or pulling too hard on the cranial nerves. So the surgeon elected to remove it bit by bit with a long, narrow instrument resembling an elongated spoon. It was slow going because of the consistency of the tumor and the necessity to work at great depths. My job was to observe and to hold retractors from time to time.

It was approaching 11 AM and more than half the tumor remained. The surgeon was consistently monitoring the clock. All of a sudden the pace of tumor removal picked up noticeably. Instead of long, slow insertions of the instrument, the surgeon started making quick thrusting movements into the depths of the opening. Pieces of tumor came out much more quickly than before. There were no more intermissions so that I could see the tumor, the brain stem, and the cranial nerves.

Towards noon the surgeon declared the tumor removed. This permitted a look inside. The tumor was indeed gone and the brain stem appeared intact. But the cranial nerves looked bedraggled and some were no longer intact. The surgeon instructed the resident to close the wound, stitch up the skin, and apply the dressing. The professor was now free to make his important appointment on time. The appointment? A tennis game.

When the operation was over and we could chat, the resident asked me if I had noticed how difficult one of the bleeders was to control. I said I had noticed. Then he asked if I knew what it was. I assumed it was one of the innumerable arteries in the neck. He said it was much more than that. It was the right vertebral artery, one of the four arteries that supply blood to the brain. The implication of his question and answer was clear: To have a noted professor of neurosurgery not know the location of the vertebral artery and to inadvertently sever it was almost unbelievable.

The patient's postoperative course in the hospital was good in all but one respect: The whole right side of her face was paralyzed. It sagged like the face of somebody who had had a severe stroke. Even with the regrowth of her hair and the best interventions of plastic surgeons, she would never again regain the radiant beauty she had when she entered the hospital. She would forever be regarded as a kind of cripple, the victim of a tumor that exacted its inevitable toll on her. Could it have been otherwise? I don't know for sure, but I do know that a misplaced sense of priorities may well have made all the difference.

Tennis, anyone?

THE WORLD'S BIGGEST ULCER

Harry was the most memorable chief surgical resident of the 20 or so that I trained under. During the three years that I was in surgical training, he outshone the rest—who were able, competent, hard-driving men for the most part—because of a combination of ingredients, both personal and professional. And he rose above his peers in seeing what others, including me, failed to see. It was a triumph for both patient and doctor.

Harry was unprepossessing to look at: He was tall, of medium build, and slightly hunched over. He sported a home-administered crew cut. The flesh-colored frames of his glasses were perched crookedly on his nose. His demeanor switched rapidly between studied concentration on the task at hand and a bemused, almost philosophic absorption with matters that he only hinted at but never fully expressed. It did not come as a surprise to learn that he was a Harvard graduate.

Harry was not entirely in his element in the operating room. He was slow but diligent. He took time to explain what he was doing to underlings like myself. He never ceased to find humor in such well-worn teaching devices as pointing out an anatomic structure during an operation and asking what it was, hinting at it by asking such questions as: What's the answer? The word "answer" was pronounced in an attempted Brooklynese accent, the hint being that the structure was the *ansa* *hypoglossi* nerve, which was in an unexpected location for embryological reasons.

The training site was one of the three teaching hospitals of the University of California San Francisco system. The Herbert C. Moffitt Hospital was a major tertiary care center that drew patients from all over Northern California, usually because their illnesses or injuries were beyond the capabilities of community hospitals and practitioners. Sometimes the patients were afflicted with rare or atypical conditions, and other times they were not responding to treatment in their communities. The irony of our training model was that we most often saw the kind of things we would probably not see again in our professional lifetimes.

In the middle of the two-month stint that Harry and I were together, a man in his mid 50s was admitted to our service with a diagnosis of peptic ulcer. He was referred by his doctors upcountry in the Sacramento Valley because he failed to respond to treatment, including an abdominal operation and careful control of his diet. I did the initial workup on the pallid, undernourished man who was writhing and moaning in pain. His history was that he had consulted his local doctors about abdominal pain, was operated on by these doctors for an ulcer, and experienced worse pain after the operation than before, even though months had passed. His local doctors reportedly accused him of not trying hard enough to aid in his own recovery by inadequately following his special diet.

The workup included x-rays of the abdomen. The contrast of the images was enhanced by a barium swallow, which would show details of the upper gastrointestinal tract.

We got to see the x-rays and the radiologist's report two days after admission, during which the patient continued to complain of intense pain, requiring large doses of morphine just to take the edge off. The x-rays revealed that the operation by his community doctors, who were not trained surgeons, had hooked up his system in the way that peptic ulcers were experimentally induced in the dog lab. Moreover, there was a very large white mass (the barium) in an area that was presumed by the radiologists and others like me to be a sort of stomach area created by the surgery. There was one dissenter from this interpretation: Harry.

Harry couldn't stop grinning. He was in his element. He had it figured out and he couldn't contain his elation. He told me to look at the x-rays again. I said that I saw the same things as before. Then he provided the explanation. The large white spot wasn't in a newly constructed stomach; it was an ulcer, a very large ulcer, indeed a huge ulcer. The upcountry hook-up had done what it was inadvertently designed to do. It had created an ulcer so large that an experienced team of radiologists hadn't even considered that as a possibility.

The re-operation proved Harry to be exactly right. The ulcer was huge. It was beginning to eat into the backbone. Harry hooked things up the right way and bypassed the ulcer. Considering the patient's condition and the length of the surgery, the operation went well. There was hope.

When I went home that night, I was anticipating a long-needed good night's sleep. This in spite of the fact that surgical residencies of the time were notorious for inducing chronic sleep deprivation. But at two AM I received a phone call. "Dr. Masters, this is Ms. Jones, the night nurse on Ward Nine. Your patient, Mr. Stone, who was operated on for an ulcer just yesterday, isn't being cooperative." Not being cooperative? What was the problem? Was the patient pulling out his intravenous line, which would be a real problem in case he needed a blood transfusion. Not at all. He was simply refusing his pain medication.

I asked the nurse what the problem was. She said that such patients always take their pain medication because the surgery is so extensive that the pain is considerable unless morphine is administered every few hours. Snappishly, I said that if she read the doctor's orders, they called for the pain medication to be administered as needed, not routinely. This seemed to relieve her anxiety only partially. Admittedly, it was an unusual case.

I saw Mr. Stone again at morning rounds. The turnaround in his status was utterly remarkable. There was a smile on his face. He was free of pain. He refused pain medication. He adjusted to getting on a normal diet in record time. He was a new man.

The rest of us learned a lot from Harry and Mr. Stone. Thinking outside the box is the current expression. That's what Harry showed us by example. Mr. Stone taught us that pain is a relative thing; take away the most intense pain, and the remaining pain may seem trivial by comparison.

Sometimes I reflect back on Harry and Mr. Stone and wonder what would've happened if Mr. Stone hadn't been referred to our training program and been assigned to such an astute surgeon as Harry. My guess is that he may well have wasted away in agony until he died a few weeks or months later. Perhaps he might have been put in contact with more capable practitioners than his doctors upcountry, but I have my doubts. For certain there was no better outcome than that afforded by Harry.

THE COLD LEG FROM OROVILLE

A glimpse of how the US Government works—or doesn't work—can be had by looking into the vast bureaucracy known as the Veterans Administration, or VA. I had the opportunity to do just that by virtue of being a University of California San Francisco surgical resident doing a training rotation at the VA hospital in San Francisco. During an aggregate period of four months of exposure to the VA from 1964 to 1966, I not only participated in the care of patients but also saw how the system was manipulated for the narrowly defined benefit of the training staff—at the expense of efficient provision of care and, ultimately, of the taxpayer.

The first realization that things were different at the VA hospital came when it became glaringly apparent that there were a number of patients who were way overdue for discharge. Some, like the young man who was a month post-operative from an uncomplicated hernia repair, pleaded to be discharged, only to be told by a staff surgeon that, no, it wasn't time yet. When would it be time? "We'll let you know" was the stock reply. The reason the patients didn't sign out against medical advice (AMA) was that they didn't want to jeopardize their status with the VA. They were captives of a sort.

When the discharge does occur, it comes when the staff surgeon suddenly decides, for no readily apparent reason, that a patient is deemed ready to go. It doesn't take long to become aware that there is a high degree of correlation between the discharge and the admission of a patient with a condition that the surgeons want to operate on.

Then the newbie trainee asks a staff member: Why the cat-and-mouse game? The staff member explains, as though for the hundredth time, that the VA regulations require such behavior because, otherwise, the bed will be filled by somebody without an operable surgical condition. The newbie slowly becomes aware that there is an army of veterans seeking admission to the VA hospital, and that almost none have conditions warranting admission to a hospital. However, the presence of an empty hospital bed creates a kind of political vacuum that sucks in whomever is highest in the pecking order at that moment. And that whomever is very likely not to contribute to the training program one iota.

Like any system, it can be gamed by outsiders, perhaps including those whose formative years were spent training in a VA hospital. I experienced such an instance when I spent the weekend on call at the San Francisco VA hospital.

I got a call from a surgical staff member one Friday evening to expect an admission in several hours. According to him, a doctor in Oroville, a town in the Sacramento Valley about 150 miles from San Francisco, had just called him concerning an urgent surgical case in a veteran. He described the patient as having just experienced a sudden blockage in the arterial circulation to one leg. Emergency vascular surgery could remove the blockage and save the leg. The case would become known as "the cold leg from Oroville."

Because the case was considered acute, an ambulance was authorized to transport the patient. The patient was received at the VA hospital with some little fanfare until a brief look by the surgical staff made them realize that they had been had. The affected leg was hot, red, and swollen, a condition that had existed for at least a week. No surgery was indicated because the condition was caused by a blocked vein, not an artery, and only standard medical treatment was required. The referring doctor's prevarication worked—he successfully dumped a patient with a medically uninteresting condition on the system. It would be a long time before the bed he occupied would become available to a so-called "interesting case."

Several years ago, around the year 2010, I was in San Francisco and decided to kill an hour between appointments by visiting the VA hospital. The original 1940s style Art Deco building was overwhelmed by add-ons on all sides. The expanded parking lot was full. There were all the signs of a bloated federal bureaucracy, local style. But one thing hadn't changed: When I ducked into a side door to use the restroom, the interior had the same drab, timeworn appearance. And the clientele in the canteen and at the bus stop had the same down-and-out appearance of people—mostly men—whose lives were filled with too much booze and too many cigarettes.

A recent discussion with a friend who had been in the same surgical training program revealed that he, too, had a memorable experience with the VA hospital system. During his first day on the surgical ward, he noticed that none of the patients required further hospitalization. And so he discharged them. The next day my friend was summoned by the chief of surgery at the VA to explain his actions. The professor ordered him to fill all the empty beds with "patients" on top of the waiting list. The rationale was that an annual audit was just a week away, and his budget would be slashed unless all the beds were full.

My friend said that he did what he was told. The beds were promptly filled with new "patients." When they made rounds the next day, the professor asked my friend the diagnosis and status of each "patient" as they passed from bed to bed. At each bed the verbal report varied only slightly from "Mr. Smith is a fifty-seven-year-old white male who has a long history of heavy cigarette smoking and chronic lung disease. He is in the hospital because there was an available bed. We are continuing the same treatment regimen that he was following before hospitalization."

After a half dozen of such reports, the professor said to my friend: "It appears that all the patients on this ward might have the same diagnosis. Is that true?" My friend answered yes. Further rounds were canceled. And my friend learned a valuable lesson: Don't try to take on the VA bureaucracy by yourself, no matter how rational your motives.

DEATH SENTENCES

They were not two of a kind, but fate had similar plans for them. Fate was especially unkind because each man had a great deal to offer the world. They had special insight into what was happening to them because both were members—especially gifted members—of the medical profession.

ⅉⅉⅉ

Eli had left New York City in 1961 for an internship at the San Francisco General Hospital, a teaching institution that was part of the University of California medical complex. Within moments after meeting him, he evoked the adage: You can take the boy out of the City, but you can't take the City out of the boy. He was loud, brash, and seemingly always in a rush, eating on the run between patients and wards. He was pudgy, balding, and sallow. He looked like he hadn't exercised a day in his life. The pockets of his white intern's jacket were stuffed with Twinkies and the like. Bagels weren't there because they were unavailable in that part of San Francisco.

Being a third-year medical student, as I was at the time, meant that you were assigned to a different service—internal medicine, surgery, obstetrics, et cetera—every few weeks in order to get a glimpse of the various medical specialties. It also meant that you were exposed to a number of interns, who were the next tier up in the medical hierarchy. In addition to taking care of patients, it was their job to teach you, and it was your job to learn from them as well as be their gofer. This is where Eli reenters the picture.

The first encounter with Eli was a little like being hit by a tornado. His first words to me, uttered in a loud rush, were "Hi, I'm Eli," pronounced as "Hoy, I'm Ee-loy." He then finished inserting a catheter into the bladder of an elderly man, showing me the tricks of the trade when it was a difficult insertion, as this one was. When his hands were busy with a procedure or writing a note in a chart, he talked nonstop, sharing his amazingly extensive knowledge of things medical.

When he was between patients and wards, he strode so fast that it took considerable effort to keep up with him. All the while he was cramming the contents of his pockets into his mouth as quickly as he possibly could. He looked like a perfect candidate for a heart attack.

The two weeks with Eli were undoubtedly the best exposure I had to clinical medicine during my student days. He seemed to have a much greater store of knowledge than his fellow interns and he was a gifted teacher. He would make a real contribution to medicine as he pursued his career.

Two months after the rotation with Eli, I was making late-afternoon rounds with the medical resident and the intern I'd been assigned to. Our first stop was the radiology department, where we looked at the x-rays taken that day. In the stack of x-rays was a chest x-ray of Eli, but no indication of why it was taken. Odd. Our next stop happened to be the cardiology lab. There, standing in the middle of the room with his shirt off and pants legs rolled up, was Eli. He held an electrocardiogram tracing in his hands and was scrutinizing it intensely. Unlike most of us at that stage of our training, Eli was perfectly capable of interpreting an EKG. He understood the message it contained: You are a dead man.

Eli was hospitalized at San Francisco General and given a private room. Five days later, the cardiology staff was making its daily rounds and stopped at Eli's room. When they knocked on the door, Eli said to give him a minute as he had to use the bedside commode. They waited a few minutes. There was no sound emanating from the room. They entered and found Eli dead of a heart attack. He was 26.

꙳꙳꙳

Hank was a medical school classmate. He was among the best students in a class of 100. He did not get the gold-headed cane at graduation, the prize awarded by the faculty for being the best all-around doctor, but I'm reasonably certain that he was a close runner-up. He was personable, always eager to learn, and had a gentle sense of humor.

He stayed at the medical center in San Francisco, trained in radiology, and was asked to join the faculty when he completed his residency. He rose through the ranks to become a full professor at what had become one of the leading medical schools in the nation.

Not only was he a gifted teacher, Hank was a devoted family man and amateur musician as well. Life was good, and he deserved it.

Being a radiology professor wasn't just a job to Hank; it was a passion. Despite the demands on him as a leading specialist in gastrointestinal radiology, he always seemed to find time to sit down with a resident and review the day's x-rays. This was not just a routine chore to Hank; this was a time to share his vast knowledge as well as to hone his skills. He was in his element.

One day a resident brought him some interesting abdominal films to read. Together, they went through each, with the resident proffering his opinion and Hank commenting on how near or far his opinion was from the resident's. Partway through the stack of x-rays, Hank saw one that instantly incited his interest, so much so that he jumped in with his own interpretation instead of waiting for the resident to go first.

One of the professional pleasures of being on the diagnostic side of medicine is to be able to make an accurate diagnosis at a glance, especially if the disease is rare. Hank was sure that he was spot-on. In front of the two was the x-ray of a classic case of a rare cancer located deep in the abdomen near the bile duct and the pancreas. Hank couldn't help but proclaim that the cancer was inoperable and the patient was doomed. Since the case was of special interest from a teaching point of view, Hank looked for the patient's name on the side of the film. He recognized it. It was his own name. He hadn't given a thought to the workup he'd gone through a few days earlier to track down the cause of vague symptoms he'd been having in recent months.

As usual, the professor was always right, at least in Hank's case. Three months after the diagnosis was made, Hank died of the rare cancer. He was 67.

Brushes with Death

One of my most cherished quotations, attributed to John Maynard Keynes, the famous English economist, is: "In the end, we're all dead." How true. And how British. As an American, I have to contend with the fact that I live in a death-denying society. An American, typically, is not as straightforward about death as are peoples from other cultures. For example, you have only to pick up a morning newspaper in the United States to find out who, during the past two or three days, has "passed away"; "gone to be with Jesus"; "met their maker"; or (my favorite) "joined the angels in heaven." I wish.

This is not to say that I am cavalier about death. I'm not, especially when it comes to my own passing. But I don't try to evade the issue by circumlocutions. Death is death, period. But what about near-death experiences? Do they not make life seem more precious, more vivid, more alive?

I myself have had several brushes with death—close calls as they say in the movies. Although they happened decades ago, each event is deeply etched in my memory, a memory that is otherwise remarkable for its ability to forget. Why this attachment to memories of brushes with death? I don't have a complete answer, but I do think it has a great deal to do with becoming hyperaware of the finality of death. There's no going back, no second chances. One realizes that, if things happened just a little bit differently, the lights would've gone out forever.

The following are seven personal accounts of brushes with death.

BREATHLESS

My first brush with death—and still the most terrifying, even though it took place over 50 years ago—was when I went stream fishing in the Sierras with a friend. One summer's day, when I was 19, Bill and I drove up from Sacramento to the stream bank at the 2,500-foot level. I decided to try my hand at spearfishing using a metal trident mounted on a five-foot pole. We had no scuba gear; we used fins and a mask instead. The water was about eight feet deep, clear and not terribly cold.

I was the first to go in. Bill waited for me on the bank. Just after entering the water, I saw a ten-inch-long fish, probably a trout, and tried to spear it. No luck. I saw it dart into the shadows under the opposite bank. As I neared the fish, I could make out that it had taken refuge in an underwater cave that extended back about eight feet. Thinking that I could improve upon my luck, I followed the fish into the cave, which consisted of a space lined by boulders. The entryway was snug but not tight. No problem, I thought. The fish evaded me, so I tried to back out. I then realized that the fins on my feet precluded backing out. Unsurprisingly, I was beginning to feel short of breath since I had only a gulp of air just before I entered the water.

At that moment I knew I was a dead man if I panicked, and probably a dead man if I did not. Such a situation wonderfully concentrates the mind. I had to get out of the cave—but how? I sensed that I had to get out head first. So I contorted my body in measured steps so that I gradually turned around. There was not an inch or a second to spare in doing so. Moments later, I surfaced, seemingly none the worse for wear. I told Bill that a few more moments of entrapment would have been fatal, and he would have had the unhappy duty to notify the authorities.

To this day I can relive every moment in the cave, and even see my drowned body being removed by a scuba diver with the Sheriff's Department.

A CHOKING SENSATION

The Mission Emergency Room of the San Francisco General Hospital was the place where second-year surgical residents like me trained in providing emergency care to whomever came through the door, usually by ambulance with sirens screaming. The ER was really a series of rooms attached to the far northern end of the hospital, near the operating rooms and the x-ray department. Central to the series of rooms was the nurses' desk, where highly experienced nurses administered the flow of patients from admission to discharge.

To staff the emergency room on a round-the-clock basis, there were two second-year surgical residents, one there for 10 hours during the day and the other during the remaining 14 hours, starting at 6 PM. They alternated shifts weekly, which not only varied the kinds of cases seen but also played havoc with their sleep-wakefulness cycle. Assisting the resident on duty were interns and medical students, but it was he (there were only he's in the mid-1960s) who supervised and decided whether the patient should be admitted, discharged, or considered for an emergency surgical operation by a fifth-year resident.

A problem arose when a patient was deemed to require care beyond acute emergency treatment. Patients who were indigent were offered follow-up treatment at the hospital or its clinics, whereas patients who were covered by medical insurance had to receive further evaluation and treatment elsewhere. During the day there were trained social workers on staff who "socialized" the patient to determine where their follow-up care might be received. At night it fell to the second-year resident to accomplish this task, something for which he was neither trained nor given guidance.

The rationale, if there ever was one, for the lack of social worker coverage at night was never given. There was no less need for socialization at night, especially when things got busy. Weekend nights after major ball games in town tended to generate more business than usual. We referred to this phenomenon as due to the weekly meeting of the knife and gun club.

The axis around which the entire ER rotated was the evening charge nurse, Mrs. Fogler. A sixtyish white-haired woman, she radiated authority. Dressed in her crisply starched white uniform and with an utterly professional demeanor, she seemed to be everywhere at once, calmly helping to restore order to an inherently chaotic mix of patients, families, doctors, nurses, ambulance drivers, orderlies, portable x-ray machines, IV poles, shrieks of pain, and moans of despair. It seemed relevant that her son was a San Francisco cop.

Usually the influx of new patients slowed to a trickle after midnight. It was then possible for the resident in charge to contemplate getting some rest and perhaps some sleep. In recognition of this the ER was lightly staffed after the evening shift. Most important, there was neither a Mrs. Fogler nor a social worker to lend their expertise when things got unexpectedly busy.

All this came to a head for me a little after midnight at a time when I had been on the ER rotation for a couple of months. Things were pretty quiet. A man in his mid 30s, accompanied by a ten-year-old girl, was waiting to talk to me after being seen by one of the staff. He said that he was seeking emergency treatment of his daughter, but was unable to convince the first doctor he saw (an intern) of this. According to him, she was seriously ill with a bad cold. She appeared to be "in no acute distress," as the medical jargon went. So I told him that, under the circumstances, she didn't warrant emergency treatment. He seemed to be quite displeased by this, and insisted that she be treated.

It was becoming apparent that the furor had more to do with personal problems within the family than with any physical illness. It seemed that the man was estranged from his wife, the girl's mother, and the father was trying in some way to show his concern about his daughter. After a quick socialization, I found out that he was a union member and therefore had health insurance. I then recommended that, if he was still concerned, he contact his doctor, if he had one. If not I would contact one for him. He opted for the latter, so I contacted a private doctor and informed him of the situation. The doctor said he would be willing to see the patient that night, if the father insisted, or he could see the patient the next day. I informed the father of this and asked him for a decision. He demurred. I said that I had other patients to attend to, and left open the option of calling the private doctor again.

I then went to the back of the nurses' station where there was a small alcove hidden by a drapery. Inside was a bathroom sink where I splashed water on my face and washed my hands. Unbeknownst to me, the father of the girl had entered the nursing station area and was waiting for me to emerge from the alcove. I told him to wait outside the nurses' station while he made up his mind about which option he wanted to pursue.

The next thing I knew, I was backed over the sink in the alcove with the father's hands on my throat. He was choking me to the point that I couldn't breathe at all. I couldn't get any leverage to push him away. Probably because the nurses' station had been empty moments before, nobody came to break us apart. I could think of only one thing to do before I passed out from lack of oxygen. It was suggested by a comic book I had read at about the age of ten. The hero overcame the attack of the villain by ejecting an eye with the flick of a finger.

I jammed my right index finger up into the inside of my attacker's left eye and pulled as hard as I could. That got his attention. He let go of my throat and then backed away from me to the point that I could stand up straight. The curtain covering the entrance to the alcove parted, and suddenly there were people pulling us apart. It was over for me and I resumed my duties.

A couple of hours later I was told that the man had been admitted to the county hospital on the ophthalmology service. He was scheduled to have surgery to repair a lacerated tear duct. My attempt to remove his eye had been unsuccessful. The comic book story didn't take into account the ligaments and other attachments that hold eyes in their sockets.

The following day I informed the chief of surgery at San Francisco General Hospital of the incident. He directed me to prepare a written account. I heard nothing further from him or any other person in an official capacity. But I did hear a few days later that my attacker was complaining to anybody who would listen about how he was the innocent victim of a white doctor in the ER.

The black and blue marks on my neck disappeared after a few weeks, and my larynx was unhurt. The attempts of my attacker to make the incident a racial issue concerned me because of the racially charged atmosphere of the mid-1960s. Scuttlebutt had it that one of my fellow surgical residents was almost sacked a couple of months earlier because of political heat over a patient who happened to be black.

I've often wondered if the emotionally charged atmosphere of the emergency room setting doesn't prompt some people to overreact. In my time stories circulated about a psychiatric resident who was shot dead by a deranged patient in the San Francisco General Hospital ER. Perhaps what happened to me was just a random event. Yet I believe that proper staffing—with 24-hour-a-day, seven-day-a-week coverage by social workers and security personnel—would likely have prevented the attack on me.

DEADLY PATHWAY

In my second tour of duty in Vietnam, in 1968–69, I was the head of a three-man US Army Special Forces (Green Beret) medical team researching rampant, disabling skin diseases among US infantrymen in the hot, humid Mekong Delta. The two sergeants and I were officially assigned to the Walter Reed Army Institute of Research in Washington, DC, but our duty station was with the US Ninth Infantry Division, which was so plagued by skin diseases that they affected the division's ability to conduct combat operations.

The division's base was in a place near the Mekong River. At Dong Tam we had a small laboratory co-located with the surgical hospital where we kept our research records and such things as the bacterial and fungal culture specimens taken from lesions on soldiers' skin. In a sense we were like any other rear area medical research unit. But we were different in that, from time to time, we visited infantry maneuver battalions in order to carry out skin disease surveys on selected infantry companies. We were then no longer in the rear area but in the forward area. In other words, we were closer to the fighting.

While this enabled us to study troops fresh from combat patrols, it did not give us firsthand knowledge of what it was like on those patrols into the swamps, paddies, and jungles. My judgment was that each research team member should accompany several patrols to get a taste of the environment in which skin diseases flourished. This, of course, would put us a lot closer to being in harm's way.

My first combat mission was with a platoon that over-nighted near the "hooch" of a Vietnamese rice farmer. We were attacked all night long, not by the Vietcong—the enemy—but by mosquitoes that thrived in paddy water. One of the men gingerly approached me, saw the insignia on the right side of my collar, and asked: "Are you a captain?" Answer: "Yes." Response: "Oh, we never see captains out here." (Their company commander was a captain.) Then he transferred his gaze to my left collar and asked: "Are you a doctor?" Answer: "Yes." Response: "Oh, wow!" I felt like a Martian intruder.

The second mission took us to a bend in a tributary of the river where we spent the night shielded by rows of Claymore mines and trip flares. No enemy river traffic was detected.

My third, and last, combat mission was with half a platoon led by a buck (lowest ranking) sergeant who seemed to have a bad attitude. We were "entrucked" to the departure point on the edge of the thick, marshy jungle. On the way, one of the junior enlisted men, a Specialist Four, made himself noticed by loudly acclaimed bravado as he faced his forthcoming task of being the point man on the patrol. The unit's mission was to penetrate and cross this area and be picked up several hours later on the other side.

After traversing an especially swampy area, where we were waist deep in water and couldn't see or hear men six feet from us due to the dense vegetation, we came upon a tiny, recently emptied hamlet hidden from aerial view by tall, shady trees. The soldiers set the bamboo hooches on fire with cigarette lighters. Two young-to-middle-aged women were trying to flee; they were captured. At the far end of the village clearing was a path back into the jungle. Just before the jungle entrance was a crudely made wooden sign with a skull and crossbones painted on it, and the message, in Vietnamese and in English, "Mortal danger. Do not proceed." We proceeded anyway along with the two women prisoners.

The path through dense jungle was so narrow that we were forced to travel single file. As it snaked along it was only possible to see one or two men in front or behind. One of the two prisoners began complaining that her knee was hurting so badly that she couldn't go any farther, and the other indicated that she needed to accompany her. The men were about to release the prisoners when it occurred to one of them that a doctor was present. I examined the allegedly afflicted woman and told the men that her knee looked perfectly all right to me. They did not release the prisoners.

Going through my mind at the time of this incident was something I had learned during my first Vietnam tour as chief of medical intelligence. A known enemy tactic was to string grenades at chest height hidden along the sides of a jungle trail and to detonate them simultaneously with a so-called command detonator. The effect was to severely damage or destroy the chest walls of their targets, after which they could easily finish off the wounded with gunfire. In our case, to kill the Americans would have resulted in the wounding or death of their women. I am virtually certain that our fate would have been sealed if the men had released the prisoners.

That the men from the village were out in the jungle ahead of us was confirmed by an incident that involved the point man, who was located a hundred or so meters ahead of me. We heard the "whump" sound of an artillery shell exploding up ahead of those of us who were located in the middle of the column. It sounded to me like a 105 millimeter artillery round. I wondered if the men had radioed our position so that we were receiving division artillery support. But there was only one round, not repeated barrages.

Moments later, a thoroughly undone point man came running back to me yelling: "Doc! Doc! Do something!" I replied that I couldn't do anything medically for him, and the fact that he was alive and not wounded or dead was worth infinitely more than anything else. The story quickly came out. At the head of the column, along with the point man, was a Tiger Scout, a Vietcong returnee to the South Vietnamese government, who recognized danger immediately ahead on the trail and restrained the point man.

Death averted by the proverbial hair.

BALING WIRE

During my research assignment in Vietnam, the three-man Special Forces research team, of which I was the head, traveled from our team base in Saigon to the US Ninth Infantry Division based in the Mekong Delta. We went out from there to several battalions belonging to the division. One was the headquarters of the 5/60th Infantry Battalion, located on the opposite side from the division of the most Vietcong-infested province in the entire Mekong Delta. It was okay to cross the river on the ferry and travel the main road in the daytime, and so we did. That trouble was not far away was proven when, in mid afternoon, US Air Force planes were laying down napalm on a grove of trees about 200 meters from the road.

We made this trip on some half dozen occasions, to and from the battalion. One mid-late afternoon we piled into the

Jeep and headed for the division's base. About a kilometer from the battalion was an enormous, flat, unvegetated area at least ten kilometers in diameter. The road went straight through this area to the river's edge where the ferry crossing was located. We got halfway across the flat area when the Jeep suddenly conked out. It wouldn't start again. The shadows were lengthening. If we walked it would be dark before we reached an American presence in either direction. We had no radio.

I had no difficulty picturing a likely scenario: Three US Special Forces soldiers, one an officer and two NCOs, were found shot to death near their Jeep in Vinh Long Province. They were apparently attacked by Vietcong forces during the night. No weapons were found but there was a partially emptied magazine of an M-16 rifle in the weeds nearby. Local villagers claim not to have seen or heard anything. Or another scenario: Three Special Forces soldiers working with the US Ninth Infantry Division have mysteriously turned up missing. Their Jeep was found along the main road in Vinh Long Province. It apparently had engine problems. The US Embassy in South Vietnam is sending a request for information about the possible capture of the soldiers by enemy forces.

The man at the wheel, Sergeant Dooley, formerly an infantryman (or "line doggie" as he termed it), now a medic, got out and raised the hood. Although he had a limited formal education, he had innate smarts and an uncanny ability to problem-solve. In ten minutes, with the equivalent of baling wire, he got the Jeep's engine to start again. We reached the last ferry across the river with just minutes to spare.

Thank you, Sergeant Dooley.

THERE IS A GOD

My brushes with death were not all personal—an especially memorable one was experienced vicariously. It took place in Colombia, South America, when I was with a six-person medical research team investigating the relationship between climate and the frequency and severity of fungal skin infections. Colombia was ideal for this kind of investigation because of its extremes of climate and its availability of suitable study populations. Its tropical location and Andes Mountains were key.

The team started its studies in the cool, temperate altiplano area near Bogotá, the capital, at 8,500 feet elevation. Then it moved to Medellín, the City of Eternal Spring, at 3,000 feet. After three weeks of work, I volunteered to check on the situation in a banana plantation town near sea level, a place that was a study site for us a couple of years previously. The rest of the team went to the seaside city of Cali for several days of R&R—rest and recuperation.

I drove my rented Jeep down the winding mountain roads till I hit the flat plains between the foot of the Andes and the jungle coastal area. At the apex of seemingly each hairpin turn was a crude wooden cross inscribed with a name and a date. Sometimes there were fresh-cut flowers at the base. Such was the means of commemorating the lives lost careening down the narrow mountain road at literally breakneck speed. Why take such obvious risks, time and again? My answer: machismo and pervasive fatalism.

I drove along the straight, paved two-lane road at 60 miles per hour. A mile ahead of me were two vehicles. As I approached them, I could see that the first was a taxi. There were three young nuns crammed into the backseat. A thick-set, middle-aged man was the driver. Ahead of the taxi was a mid-sized dump truck. Through the haze in the distance I could see a large vehicle coming toward us.

I decided that I had enough time to pass the taxi and truck before the oncoming vehicle was too close. So I floored the accelerator pedal and passed them. By this time the oncoming vehicle—a bus with a load of passengers—was speeding toward us. I checked the rearview mirror. To my amazement, I saw the taxi pull out into the other lane in order to pass the truck. The oncoming bus did not slow down or swerve. The taxi didn't have enough speed to pass the truck. By the time the taxi driver decided to drop back, the bus had already arrived. I heard the sound of the crash. Should I turn around to see the grisly results? No. As interesting as it might be to see what happened, I would be unable to assist the injured to any degree. Moreover, especially because of my limited Spanish, I would be unable to defend myself if the mood of the survivors turned ugly and there was an obvious scapegoat available—me, the foreigner, the gringo.

I drove toward my destination for 15 minutes; then, overcome with curiosity as to what exactly had happened in the crash, I turned around and headed back. There were no flashing lights of police cars or ambulances, probably reflecting what a remote location we were in. As I got closer to the scene, I saw that the bus was on the right shoulder of the highway and was missing its left front wheel. Passengers were slowly and resignedly filing out of it. Opposite the bus, the taxi driver, dripping blood from the superficial cuts on his face, neck, and torso, was staggering in front of his cab. In the backseat, apparently unharmed physically, were the three sisters, sitting bolt upright and mute in their blue nuns' habits. They clearly had seen the face of their god.

Looking more closely at the taxi, I saw that the hood and engine were missing. The engine block was located 150 feet away in a field. The bus must have hit the angled cab in just such a way as to apply all the force in shearing off the engine rather than crushing the engine into the passenger compartment.

As I left the scene for the second time, I wondered: blind fate or divine intervention? Whatever the answer, I was sure of at least one thing: Hispanic machismo is a curse of that culture. I was reasonably certain that the taxi driver attempted to pass the truck because he couldn't stand the idea of a foreigner—a gringo—making him feel unmanly.

AT GUNPOINT

In the early 1980s I was stationed at the Presidio of San Francisco and had an apartment on Russian Hill that offered an unobstructed view of the Bay Bridge and the sparkling lights of the East Bay. It was a posh part of town, just above the Art Institute. Further on were Ghirardelli Square and Coit Tower.

One Thursday evening I was invited to dinner in Sausalito by a former girlfriend. During dinner we reminisced over a bottle of wine. Since the following day was a work day, I left Sausalito just after 10 PM. Twenty minutes later I was in front of the door to the basement garage of my apartment building, and pushed the door opener button in my car, a little Fiat X1/9 hardtop convertible. The door slowly opened, as usual, and I drove in, turned left, and parked in my assigned space.

When I stepped out of my car, I noticed some unexpected movement at the corner of my right eye, and made a startled "ugh" sound. An instant later two men wearing stocking masks confronted me from two to three feet away. One pointed a nickel-plated revolver at me and then instructed me to spread-eagle over my car door. Before I complied, I tried doing some quick computations in my head using Bayes' theorem, a several-centuries-old formula for calculating the probability of an event—such as being shot in the head—given a particular set of circumstances. My mental computer didn't work optimally; undoubtedly the combination of the wine and the surprise didn't help. Reverberating in my head was the question: What gives me the best chance of survival? To comply with their instructions? Or, if they plan to shoot me after robbing me, try to kick the gun away? There were two of them and only one of me, and they had the gun. Also, they appeared to be strong, stocky men in their thirties. Bad odds. But going through my head was a front-page news story the previous week that described a daytime armed robbery of a candy store in San Francisco in which the two masked male robbers gratuitously shot three people dead. Were these the same robbers? Would they kill me even if I complied with everything they asked?

I decided to go spread-eagled over my car. They stripped me of my wallet, a keychain, and gold watch. After asking how they could open the garage door for their departure, they ordered me to lie facedown on the garage floor and slowly count to 100. This was my last chance to wrest the gun away.

The odds seemed overwhelmingly in their favor, so I complied. I fully anticipated hearing a loud noise followed by utter silence and complete blackness.

By the time I counted to ten, I could hear them going to the garage door, and at 25 I got up from the floor. To my surprise my legs were not shaking. I calmly walked toward the inside door to the apartment building, along the way picking up my keychain and empty wallet. Upon reaching my apartment, I called 911 and reported the incident. Twenty minutes later, an old, beat-up car arrived noisily outside the building. A minute later, two young plainclothes cops—the Mod Squad less Linc, the black guy—appeared at my apartment door. I told them what had happened. They said they would file a report and that would probably be the end of it. When I expressed my frustration at this outcome, one of them said: "Look, sir, you're lucky. Three weeks ago, just a block up the hill from here, a retired lawyer in his seventies, who tried to resist a similar robbery, was pistol-whipped by two men so badly that he's still in the hospital because of head injuries."

What did I take away from this experience?

- Crime does pay, much more often than we're led to believe by lifelong propaganda that "crime doesn't pay."

- If screened to serve as a juror in a criminal trial, I would probably be excused forthwith when my decidedly Old Testament views, influenced by personal experience with criminals, were expressed.

- Powerful visions of what I would do to the two men if I had the gun and they were at my mercy. There would be no mercy. They would be sitting facing each other at an angle, bound and gagged with their eyes taped open. The rest I leave to your imagination.

- A profound sense of violation. For this reason, this kind of crime is, to my mind, a wholly different thing from "victimless crime," such as using currently illicit drugs or engaging in prostitution.

BLACK ICE

One of the duties of the senior specialist physician assigned to a major headquarters in the Army is to make consultant visits to corresponding specialists in the headquarters catchment area. In my case, I was stationed in San Antonio, Texas, and was the consultant in preventive medicine. In midwinter in early 1980, I was called upon to visit Fort Carson, Colorado, just outside Colorado Springs, about 60 miles south of Denver.

After flying to Denver I spent the night there and woke the next day to find that there had been a light snowfall. I called the state highway patrol and was told that the interstate between Denver and Colorado Springs was open. So I started driving south in my economy rental car. The day was gray and cloudy but clear, and the drive was initially uneventful. On the highway, my initial cruising speed was 40 miles per hour. Because there seemed no reason not to, the speed crept up to 65 to 70 miles per hour.

Only in retrospect did I realize that I had been on a several-miles-long, gradual rise. At the end of the rise, the highway unexpectedly made a sharp descent. Suddenly I no longer had any control of the car. The brakes and steering wheel were useless. The car was headed to the outer part of the divided highway at 70 miles per hour. It was then that I noticed the aluminum light stanchions at 50-foot intervals along the side of the highway. It was obvious that if a car hit a light stanchion, there would be only one winner—and it wasn't the car. I experienced a quiet realization that the car and I were entirely in the hands of fate, that we would perish or survive together.

Somehow—somehow—the car stopped at the side of the highway, the two right-side wheels in a ditch. The tow truck arrived an hour later. The car, not to mention the driver, was unhurt. The rest of the trip was at a snail's—nay, a tortoise's—pace. I arrived at Fort Carson in the afternoon rather than the morning, after a very slow rest of the journey.

At 4 PM, it was time to go back to Denver before it got too dark. I remained a tortoise, never exceeding 30 miles per hour. My fellow northbound travelers whizzed past me, usually with a sneer if not with their noses totally in the air. About 20 minutes into the trip, I saw a half-mile ahead of me that a car in the left lane suddenly veered left onto the divider strip. Then another and another. Passing strange. Were they having a conclave? When I came abreast, I could see one of the drivers in the parallel line of cars. His face was immobile, ashen gray, and had a wide-eyed stare, as though he had looked death in the face. The hares had seen their maker, and were speechless.

Funny what a patch of black ice can do to a person.

COOLING OFF

Some brushes with death may be more in the mind than in physical reality. I experienced just such a phenomenon when I developed heart trouble while stationed at the US Army hospital in Landstuhl, Germany. It was early in the year 1984 and I had just turned 46. I had felt peculiar sensations in my chest and discovered that my heartbeat was irregular.

Soon after visiting the cardiologist, I found myself hospitalized in the cardiac care unit and assigned a single room. I was monitored electronically after electrocardiograph leads were pasted on my body. I was given the standard cardiac patient's diet—tasteless, whitish muck intended to reverse a lifetime of overeating fatty foods by cholesterol-plaque-prone patients. It didn't seem to matter that I was in good physical shape, ate sensibly, exercised regularly, and did not have coronary artery disease. Passed without notice was that, during the previous few months, I was under extreme stress as a result of being trapped in a brief, unfortunate marriage.

The hospital room was stark white: walls, floor, and ceiling. The hospital buildings dated from World War II when the Germans used them for their troops. My room was utterly bare except for the bed and a portable white privacy screen on one side near the back. In short, Kafka-esque.

As night came on, I felt chilled so I pulled the lightweight bedcovers up around me. That sufficed temporarily. Some hours later, I woke in the dark and felt extremely cold. Since I was in one of the Army's leading hospitals, and in the special care unit, I assumed that the cold I felt must be the result of my medical condition. So I said to myself: *This must be what it feels like to die over a several-hour period. One simply cools off till it's over.*

I was still alive and conscious the next morning when a nurse came into my room. I told him what I had been experiencing. He agreed that the room felt quite cold. He then looked around for the cause. Could it be something like a blocked heating duct? To examine the room thoroughly, he moved the portable privacy screen from against the wall. There was the answer. Just above the baseboard was a 6 x 12 inch rectangular hole in the wall that communicated with the outside, which was freezing cold. I was then transferred to a different room, which was suitably warm. No more death thoughts.

I've since wondered what I'd find if I returned to that hospital's cardiac care unit. Would I find a privacy screen still hiding the hole in the wall? It wouldn't surprise me.

Join the Army and...

Seeing the world wasn't what I had in mind when, in 1966, I volunteered to go into the Army in order to get my two-year military obligation out of the way. I was then an "obligated volunteer," obligated to go where I was sent by what was informally known as the Green Machine. Despite attempts to spend my service time in Europe or Hawaii, I was sent to Vietnam in order to help President Lyndon Johnson "nail the coon skin on the wall." We failed, as everybody knows.

The year in Vietnam wasn't entirely ill-spent. My assignment was in medical intelligence. Since nobody in Vietnam seemed to know what that was, I could travel around South Vietnam largely as I pleased. I went as far north as Da Nang, where I saw the US Marines tie themselves up in knots, and as far south as Phu Quoc Island, where junior US naval officers got drunk and fought each other once a week simply to let off steam. But overall, Vietnam was a beautiful country, even in wartime.

For the first four months, my intelligence unit was co-located with a medical research team from the Walter Reed Army Institute of Research (WRAIR, as in "rare"). The team was involved in studying diseases of military importance, especially those in the tropics. I became interested in joining the Special Forces (Green Beret) component of the team, even at the expense of throwing away the three arduous years I'd spent in surgical training prior to joining the Army.

When the year in Vietnam was up, I found myself jumping out of planes flying over Georgia, Alabama, and North Carolina, slogging through the Florida Everglades, and returning to Vietnam to conduct research in the Mekong Delta. I was hooked.

The next thing I knew, I was a resident trainee in preventive medicine at the WRAIR headquarters in Washington, DC. In three years I investigated epidemic-related diseases in Colombia, Panama, and Texas. Three years after that, when I was stationed at the Letterman Army Institute Research in San Francisco, I participated in studies in Alaska and again in Colombia. During those six years I presented the results of our studies in places as far away as Brazil.

As I was learning about the Army, the Army was learning about me. Early on, when I was selected for unappetizing temporary assignments while more senior colleagues were sent to relative garden spots, I was told that this was in keeping with longstanding custom. In later years when I had become much more senior, I was selected to go to such places as the scorching deserts of Saudi Arabia in midsummer. The rationale given was that, by virtue of my extensive experience, I was especially suited for the challenging task at hand. It finally dawned on me that the people making the assignments viewed me as being made up of much more pliable material than my colleagues. By that time, it was too late. But in the interim I found that your reputation precedes you (not always a bad thing) and hard-won experience leaves an indelible mark (not always a bad thing either).

What follows are accounts of travel to parts of the world ranging from Saudi Arabia in the summer to northern Alaska in the winter. The travel was disguised as work.

COLOMBIA

Colombia, South America, is not for the faint of heart. It is a land of extremes, which is the reason we were there. We needed the extremes of climate for our research into their effects on the rate and severity of common skin infections. We didn't need the extremes of poverty and wealth nor the imminent threats of violence that are the country's legacy; they came with the package. Included was an incredible amount of geographic diversity within an area eight times smaller than the United States: a bone-dry desert and a 21,000-foot-high snowcapped mountain right next to the ocean; lowland jungles harboring monkeys and malaria within easy driving distance from a major metropolis in a balmy climate; the dusty, sere high plains—the *Altiplano*—of the interior; and above all the jagged peaks of the Andes Mountains.

By we, I mean Professor Damon Tarpin of the University of Miami School of Medicine and myself, an Army medical officer from the Walter Reed Army Institute of Research in Washington. We had worked collaboratively on epidemic skin diseases among American troops in the Vietnam War several years previously and found ourselves in a position to work together again. We were assisted by a research associate from Miami and two Colombian physicians.

A month after receiving the invitation phone call from Damon in 1971, I was headed to Bogotá, the capital city, located at 8,500 feet in the Altiplano, where the night chill was warded off by colorful wool garments akin to Mexican *serapes*. Damon had reserved a room for me at the Tequendama Hotel, the poshest place in town. It was amazingly affordable because of favorable currency exchange rates. At Damon's urging, I had a manicurist do my fingernails. Then we had cocktails in the dimly lit bar where the bartender wore a cape and swirled around to wait on customers. Later, we were greeted by the attendant at the elevator with the phrase *a la orden* (to your order). It was pure luxury.

Two days later the fairy tale ended. We began our surveys of schoolchildren in orphanages around the Bogotá area. Their accommodations were extremely modest by American standards. I came to regret the manicure not only because the cuticle was removed to the point of lingering painfulness but also because my highly polished fingernails seemed so out of place in the face of such poverty.

Unlike the United States, with its so-called inner cities, the slums of South America are located on the outskirts, often on steep hillsides with no electricity or running water. They are usually populated by impoverished *campesinos*, country people who leave the agricultural countryside for life in the city. I prevailed upon a couple of our Colombian hosts to take me to see a typical example of life in the slums. I was taken to a room in a ramshackle hillside building where the occupant was a gray-haired woman whose family had deserted her. She took her meals of beans and rice from a heavily dented aluminum pot that was encrusted with the remains of previous meals. She had no means of washing the pot and spoon. She slept on the floor atop a tattered pile of sheets and blankets. There was no furniture other than a wobbly wooden chair. It was a reminder that, in countries like Colombia, the rates and degrees of poverty—true poverty—are staggering compared to those in the US.

Our next stop was Medellín at 3,000 feet, just enough altitude to create a springtime environment despite the fact that it is just a few degrees north of the equator. Beautiful flower gardens were everywhere. We surveyed children at nearby orphanages and found that, in sanitary conditions similar to those in Bogotá, more of the children had bacterial skin infections, presumably related to the warmer climate.

Our trip was not all work and no play. We seized opportunities for diversion as they arose. For example, while on an errand I was driving on a major road on the outskirts of town. I noticed a large sign with letters proclaiming: *Fresas con Crema* (strawberries with cream). I decided to return that afternoon. Though I'm not a strawberry devotee, I was captivated by the luscious ripeness of the berries and the perfection of the whipped cream. Superb. And the garden in which they were served made me realize why Medellín was called, lovingly, the City of Eternal Spring. The drug lords who moved in a decade later certainly picked well in terms of a garden spot in which to conduct their business.

A short distance from Medellín was a Colombian army encampment at the same altitude but in a drier environment. We surveyed troop units and found skin infections at a little lower rate than in the children.

We drove down the mountains to a warm, moist, tropical area near the Panamanian border. We stayed at a small banana plantation town called Apartado, where there was basic lodging. There was a dusty main road through the center of town that was lined on both sides for three blocks by bars and brothels. A number of the men wore revolvers on their hips. It was raw and reminiscent of small frontier towns in the Western US in the 1880s.

The orphaned children we surveyed had a much higher rate of skin infections, presumably reflecting the higher number of mosquito bites, among other things. Soldiers just back from a combat mission against insurgents in the jungle had the highest skin infection rates of all. Almost a third were affected.

To provide medical services to the region around Apartado, the Colombian government had established a hospital staffed by recent medical school graduates. They were performing their required two years of national service. There were no older, more experienced doctors available. We talked to them and were impressed by both their knowledge and their devotion to the care of their patients. They performed surgery, sometimes of a very advanced kind, because there was no one else to do it.

At the time of our visit, they had a young man who had sustained massive trauma to his torso and was bleeding profusely into his urinary tract from a ruptured kidney. To save his life it was necessary to control the bleeding by an operation to remove the damaged kidney, leaving the other one to carry on its vital functions. But what if the patient had the rare condition known as "horseshoe kidney," in which the two kidneys were fused together before birth? The young doctors' primitive x-ray machine showed that there was indeed a horseshoe kidney, and therefore it was necessary to attempt to leave the intact half of the kidney in the patient. Despite heavy odds against it, the attempt was successful. Who would've expected such an outcome in this remote area of the world?

We returned to Bogotá to prepare our equipment and laboratory specimens for shipment. The study had gone well. Just before noon on a main road on the outskirts of Bogotá, we noticed a large building on our left. Damon asked: "Isn't that the Army headquarters?" I confirmed that it was the Colombian equivalent of the Pentagon. Damon insisted on stopping and offering a briefing on skin diseases in the troops we had surveyed. I said it sounded like a crazy idea to me. Imagine what would happen to foreigners in the US who got it into their minds to barge into the Pentagon and ask to brief the top-ranking officer.

We entered the lobby of the headquarters, looked around, and were asked, in Spanish, what we were looking for. Seeing that we were not fluent, we were guided to a sharp-looking lieutenant colonel who spoke excellent English. He looked puzzled when we admitted we didn't have an appointment, and perplexed when we said we'd like to brief the top general. He very politely said he'd check to see if the general was available. To his (and my) amazement, he was. The officer politely excused himself. We were on our own.

After waiting 45 minutes, we were summoned into the top general's office. We took a seat at one end of the extremely spacious room, were served the obligatory coffee, and looked up at the other end of the room when the general entered. He appeared to be well into his sixties if not early seventies. We asked if he spoke English; he said none. No interpreter was present. He asked why we had asked to see him. I looked over at Damon and waited for him to respond. He just sat there with an embarrassed smile on his face.

Without moving my lips I said, "*Damon*. This was your idea, wasn't it? Please speak up." Not a word from him. I couldn't stand the silence any longer, so I delivered an impromptu briefing in my halting Spanish. The general seemed satisfied. I had survived yet another surprise by my professor friend.

Damon reworked my trip report and submitted it to *The Lancet*, a prominent British medical journal. It was published as a lead article. That in itself made it a worthwhile trip; but that was not all. We had lingering memories of the somber beauty of Colombia. In contrast with Mexico, the color seemed less bright, the music more subdued, and the people more restrained. There was a haunting quality that made us want to return.

In 1974 I found myself back in Colombia as a member of a joint US Army-University of Miami research team whose mission was to study fungal skin infections in geographically diverse parts of the country. The team's goal was to replicate the study on bacterial skin infections that some of us had carried out two years previously, but this time to study fungal skin infections.

Upon landing in Bogotá, the country's capital, it became apparent that security was even tighter than during the previous trip. The airport was crawling with uniformed men—police and soldiers—armed with machine pistols. The city streets revealed the same phenomenon. To a man, their fingers were on the triggers of their weapons.

Once we found our hotel, some of us went out into the downtown street to see what was going on. At that moment a group of racing bicyclists swept past us. A large crowd had assembled to watch. Policemen wielded large nightsticks— clubs really—to keep the watchers off the street and on the crowded sidewalks. To enforce their commands to keep out of the street, the police raised their so-called riot batons just at the junction of sidewalk and street and slammed them downward at full force. The power of the blow would easily crack a head or break an arm. The Colombians did not seem fazed in the least by the police actions. They seemed to expect it.

On seeing this, I reflected on what I had learned about Colombia during and after the previous trip. Perhaps more than any other Latin American country, Colombia had a history and culture of violence. It was a way of life. While much of the rest of the world in the 1940s was engaged in World War II, Colombia was embroiled in turmoil because of repeated armed clashes between the Right and the Left, known as *La Violencia*. Struggle had continued in one form or another until the present day. Historians could look at it from a larger perspective: What is now called Colombia was at the center of the colonies that fought to break away from Spain in the 19th century under the leadership of the famed liberator, Simón Bolívar.

The team began its studies among army units on the outskirts of Bogotá in the cool Altiplano. As expected, few of the soldiers had fungal skin infections. But driving through the countryside to get to the units was a reminder of how somber it could be. People traveled on foot, old buses, or horses, most of whom seemed to be little more than bones and hide. The skies were cloudy and gray.

The team's next destination was Medellín, the City of Eternal Spring, and the future home of the Medellín drug cartel. We surveyed army units in the area at some length since some were stationed in arid areas and others in moister areas. Although they all resided in areas at an altitude of 3,000 feet, the rates and severity of fungal infections were not much different from those in Bogotá at 8,500 feet, or from one another.

After three weeks of arduous work, the team decided to take a break and descended on the seaside resort town of Cartagena for three days of R&R. I decided to go on my own to the banana plantation town of Apartado to check it out for a visit. It was cool and overcast. It looked even less inviting than on our visit two years earlier.

I wandered around the town. It was fiesta time in celebration of the birthday of their patron saint. But nobody seemed festive. I noticed a large dump truck parked on a side road just as it crossed the main street. A knot of people was gathered at the left rear tire. One at a time, they took turns climbing up the tire so they could see what was in the bed of the truck. I asked a policeman standing idly nearby what the people were looking at. He replied: "*Un muerto*," a dead one. Hearing this, I had to have a look for myself.

I climbed up and saw what had attracted such curiosity. Lying supine on the truck bed was the body of a laborer dressed in his work clothes and knee-length rubber boots. His head was almost completely severed from his body, being held only by a sliver of skin and underlying muscle at the back of his neck. He looked to be in his twenties or thirties, and his face was a dark reddish purple.

I climbed back down and asked what had happened. The story came out. It was fiesta time; he and a fellow laborer got drunk; a fight erupted over a woman; and one of the two was faster with his carefully honed machete than the other. The policeman did not seem particularly concerned; he just shrugged as if this was just a routine matter. The remains would probably be dumped into a pauper's grave. Life and death in the Third World.

The rest of the team and I returned to Bogotá, where we picked up supplies. We then flew to Medellín to continue studies we had initiated a couple of weeks before. One of the Miami researchers, Fran, was seated next to me. I sat next to the window, while the aisle seat on the propeller-driven plane was occupied by a Colombian mother holding an infant in a blanket. The other team members were scattered among the seats in the 80-passenger plane.

The 45-minute afternoon flight was uneventful until we reached Medellín. Like many other Andean cities, the airport was situated in a bowl in the mountains. Rain clouds hovered over the bowl, whose sides were made of jagged peaks of near-vertical granite. The plane circled round and round, looking for a break in the clouds so we could land. Looking out the cabin window, it seemed as though the wingtip was just inches away from scraping the mountain wall. Suddenly there was a small commotion in the aisle. Ordinarily fatalistic Colombians were on their knees moaning and praying. I heard utterances from the woman who was sitting next to Fran. A couple of minutes later Fran said that the woman wanted to say something to me. I told her no; when she says Señor, she means the one with the capital S, the Lord, not me, a mere señor. Moments later, the woman on the aisle handed her baby to Fran, got out of her seat, joined the other passengers kneeling in the aisle, and implored her god to save them. The prayers must have worked because five minutes later there was a hole in the clouds and we had an uneventful landing.

We drove our Land Rovers to our next soldier survey location, Barrancabermeja, in the hot, humid Magdalena River Valley. The army was there for two reasons: first, to guard the oil fields from rebel attack, and second, to mount infantry operations against the FARC guerrillas in the thick jungle of the area. These were small-unit operations with few casualties on either side. Seen in historical context, they were a continuation of the decades-old conflict between the Right and the Left.

Our survey revealed that the soldiers in the hot, humid river valley had more fungal skin infections than soldiers in cooler climates, but they were not nearly as common and severe as in US soldiers fighting in the wet lowlands of Vietnam. The climates were similar, but the exposure to a wet environment was much more common and prolonged in Vietnam.

We finished our survey and flew to Bogotá to prepare for our return to the US. The Colombian experience was not yet over.

I had heard stories about Colombia being the crime capital of the world. There were said to be schools for thieves. In my view, I had nothing to steal so I did not worry. One day, while stopped at a traffic light on a downtown Bogotá street, I was resting my left elbow on the open window frame. I was in the lane nearest the traffic island upon which stood a half-dozen people. One stepped out to beg; I ignored him. I felt him poke my arm, or so I thought. The next thing I knew, he had unstrapped my gold watch from my wrist in such a way that I barely felt it. I saw him in my rearview mirror as he escaped between me and the car behind. My only regret was that I was not quick enough to throw my vehicle in reverse and pin him against the car behind me. I would have liked to congratulate him on his excellence of technique before I turned him over to the police.

When I rejoined the other team members later in the day, they told me of the two fatalities they had witnessed while sipping drinks on the terrace at a downtown hotel. The first occurred when a young man was hit by a car when he tried to dart across a busy street. He was instantly rendered decerebrate, a type of severe brain injury, and made characteristic jerking moments before falling to the pavement while life ebbed away. Nobody stopped; they just drove around his body. Nearby was a small, upscale hotel with a sizable enclosed area between the front door and the street. An armed guard was on duty. A thief ran out of the front door trying to escape. Without hesitation, the guard shot him dead in the fenced area. The traffic kept on flowing.

We had completed our surveys within the month allotted. It was time to fly back to the US to analyze the surveys and complete the laboratory work. From the moment of landing, frenetic Miami seemed like an oasis of calm compared to daily life—and death—in Colombia.

BRAZIL

Medical mycology, the study of fungi that can cause disease in humans, is a surprisingly small field of specialization. In fact, there is only a handful of medical mycologists worldwide, and they all appear to know one another on a first-name basis. I was introduced to this select group when I was invited to present a scientific paper at the International Conference on Medical Mycology held in São Paulo, Brazil, in 1972.

My involvement in medical mycology began three years earlier when I participated in studies of skin infection epidemics among American soldiers in Vietnam. The most common and disabling type of infection in the soldiers was caused by a ringworm fungus. My co-investigator and mentor, Professor Damon Tarpin of the University of Miami, Florida, provided direction and laboratory support for the studies. He had already established himself as an authority in medical mycology and therefore was in a position to get me invited to present the paper on the results of our Vietnam studies.

At the time I was a major in the US Army Medical Corps stationed at the Walter Reed Army Institute of Research (WRAIR) in Washington, DC. The Institute, which provided authorization and funding for the trip to São Paulo, decided that it would be a good idea for me to stop off at the city of Belem at the mouth of the Amazon River on the way to São Paulo. The purpose was to visit the WRAIR (pronounced "rare") contingent of tropical medicine researchers stationed there and to assess the Amazon basin as a place to study tropical skin infections. Another consideration was that I might be stationed in Belem sometime in the future, perhaps as the team chief.

I spent the first two days in Belem before heading out for a trip west on the trans-Amazon Highway. Dinner was taken at the Brazilian officers' club along the banks of one of the mouths of the Amazon. Looking along the riverbank revealed hundreds, if not thousands, of pairs of the reddish eyes of rats reflecting boat and street lights.

My three colleagues from the WRAIR team and I set out from Belem in a Land Rover. Virtually from the outset the trans-Amazon Highway was nothing more than a red-dirt road south of the Amazon River. Soon we were enveloped in the Green Hell where, instead of the lush tropical paradise I half expected, there was just the endless monotony of un-differentiated green. The only break in the silence was from exotic birdcalls and the haunting sounds of invisible howler monkeys. Fortunately, they were far enough away that they could not throw their feces at us from the treetops.

We were south of the equator by only a few degrees. It was the dry season, so we did not have to contend with mud filling the ruts in the road. With one exception, we stayed in small, functional hotels along the way in such towns as Altamira, Maraba, and Itaituba. The exception was the night we spent in a government camp and slept in jungle hammocks.

The first evening on the road, we ate in a restaurant that specialized in meat. We were given wooden trenchers. The waiter carried a sword laden with four different meat roasts in his left hand and a dagger-like knife in his right. He then went to the man sitting to the left of me and, without warn-ing, quickly turned the sword upside down and put the point in the middle of the man's trencher. The man was then asked from which slab of meat he would like slices. It was that way all around the table. I stopped worrying about getting stuck by the sword and concerned myself instead with the deftness of the waiter. It was sheer gluttony.

Two nights later we were at the government camp. We ate out of tin cans because there were no restaurants in that remote location. It got dark right after we had eaten, so we decided to turn in early because there were no electric lights. As usual, we were covered by clinging red dust, which we did our best to remove each night before going to bed. We stripped naked and, with the aid of flashlights, strode a quarter-mile to a pond-like extension of a river tributary. The water was three to four feet deep with a diameter of 25 feet. For some reason we were not bothered by mosquitoes. However, we noticed the eyes of caymans, a kind of small alligator, at a dozen places on the shore. I kept wondering if one might be in the water and take a bite from an extremity, including male genitalia, thinking it might be a fish. We were spared.

The jungle hammocks we slept in that night had a waterproof top and sides of mosquito netting. They also contained a blanket as well as a sheet. It came as a surprise that it got noticeably cooler at night even though we were at sea level and on the equator.

The next day we had to cross the Xingu River, a major tributary of the Amazon, in order to continue on our way west. There was no bridge, only a ferry that was intermittent. We had a two-hour wait. We decided it might be entertaining as well as cooling to go swimming in the interim. The current was not strong, so it appeared safe. One of the group volunteered that piranha fish were not a problem in this part of the river; they were upstream a couple of kilometers. After we swam, the same person said the problem here was a fresh-water sponge that shed barbed spicules that entered the eye and caused blindness. They could not be removed because of the barb; they only inextricably worked their way into the eye. However, the spicules were only shed during the mating season, and this was not it. Something to keep in mind for the future.

Later that day we spotted a strange kind of animal up ahead trying to cross the road. It was moving very slowly. It was about the size of a dog, had long arms ending in three long, thick claws, and had short, greenish-brown fur. We had run across a three-toed sloth, a creature that ordinarily spends its life hanging suspended from a limb in a tall tree. Because it shyly cast its eyes downward, it reminded me of the cartoon character Mr. Magoo. We put it into the space between the back hatch and the rear seat of the Land Rover, along with a thick, three-foot stick to cling to. Nobody quite knew what to do with it, but at least it did not offer any resistance.

The next day the sloth was still there. As we rode along, hour by hour, a vision came to me. It was of Steve, who was sitting in the rear seat. He had not said anything for hours. I turned and saw a long, hairy arm around Steve's neck. Trying to arouse Steve was an impossible task. The sloth had gotten its revenge. It was then that my vision was replaced by the pleasant reality that Steve was fine and the sloth remained sloth-like, quietly holding his stick with its front claws.

Further along the way we ran across a clearing where a noticeably thin couple was in the process of trying to estab-lish a farm. They had transferred here as part of a government scheme to help the people from the impoverished northeast of Brazil. Apparently, no one had told them that, however thick the jungle, the top soil was extremely thin and would be worn out after two or three years of farming. The couple was destined to remain impoverished.

After we had spent five days going 400 miles west of Belem, it was time for me to return. I flew back in a prop plane in a couple of hours. As we neared the city, I looked out the window and saw the biggest river I had ever seen. It was enormous. I was later to learn it was only one of the five mouths of the Amazon, and that the mud it brought down from the western highlands could be seen 50 miles off the edge of the continent. It was larger by water flow than the next seven largest of the world's rivers combined.

The conference in São Paulo went as expected for such meetings. The remarkable thing was the hustle and bustle of the city itself. There was a vibrancy among the people that, if it ever existed in the US, had been nearly totally lost. I got a sense of a people who looked forward to exploiting every resource and opportunity at hand, whether it be timber and mining interests in the Amazon basin or factories in cities like São Paulo. Another striking thing: There were no apparent color barriers. People of every gradation of skin color strolled hand in hand, chatting animatedly about their lives.

The story did not end there. In the government camp we had run across three graduate students doing field research in the Amazon basin. One was a first-generation Cuban-American from Miami. She was working on a project relating to the newly established discipline of medical sociology. I told her that I had a colleague in Miami who might be interested in her field. She contacted Professor Tarpin when she returned to Miami. They hit it off and became fast friends. I received an unexpected telephone call three months after my trip to Brazil. The first voice on the line was that of a woman with a slight Spanish accent. She said, "Remember me?" How could I not?

ALASKA

In the 1970s the US Army had a considerable presence in Alaska because it was there that it was best positioned to counter aggression from the communist countries bordering the northern Pacific Ocean. The chief drawback to being stationed there was the bitter winter cold where mere freezing temperatures were nothing compared to thermometer readings of minus 50 degrees Fahrenheit. Military operations were critically dependent on protective items of uniform, particularly those to protect fingers and toes from frostbite.

To protect the feet, the US military had developed a special boot made up of layers of interior padding surrounded by a waterproof, rubberized plastic exterior. The boots were bulky and white, making the wearer look like a cartoon character. They soon acquired the sobriquet "Mickey Mouse boots." They proved remarkably effective in preventing frostbite. But the question arose: Were they too good? Might not they create a warm, humid (i.e., tropical) microenvironment and therefore be conducive to the kind of foot problems that plagued US infantrymen in Vietnam during the 1960s?

The logical place to refer such questions was the Dermatology Research Division of the Letterman Army Institute of Research in San Francisco, California. Although the US Army does not always act logically, in this case it did.

The Dermatology Research Division was tasked to answer the questions about the Mickey Mouse boots, also known as bunny boots. The tasking landed on my desk because I had conducted studies of foot and related skin problems among infantrymen in the Mekong Delta of Vietnam in the late 1960s. The date was February 1974, just in time to get to Alaska while it was still very cold.

Walt, the research chemist who accompanied me, and I boarded a commercial airliner bound for Fairbanks by way of Anchorage. Our stopover in Anchorage allowed us to deplane and walk around the airport. There, in its own separate room, was a polar bear in a metal cage. The bear was standing upright and looked to be about nine feet tall. It was simply enormous. Its thick white fur rippled on its body. Its claws were long and black. I pressed my back to the wall as I walked around the cage. I felt as though the bear could suddenly thrust its paw through the bars of the cage and impale an unfortunate gawker like me with its claws. I couldn't imagine encountering such a creature in the wild. It was completely awe-inspiring.

When we landed in Fairbanks, which is located in the middle of the state, we were told that we were lucky. The temperature the day before had gone down to minus 50 degrees, but that day it warmed up to minus 30 degrees.

The moment we stepped off the plane, we started coughing because the air was so cold and dry. The persistent coughing made it difficult to unload our scientific gear from the cargo hold of the plane. We were assisted by a representative from nearby Fort Wainwright, who promptly issued us a vital part of the winter-issue uniform. It was a heavy parka with attached mittens and a fur-lined hood. A heavy canvas strap ran through the sleeves to attach the mittens. Overkill? Not if you believe in the admonition: Lose a mitten, lose a hand.

No sooner had Walt and I arrived at Fort Wainwright's medical facility than we were informed that we had dinner invitations to the homes of the preventive medicine unit's officers for every night of our weeklong visit. When we said we didn't want to impose and might enjoy a little freedom in the evenings, it quickly became apparent that each invitation was in effect a command. It didn't make any difference that I outranked all the officers there. The unspoken message was: "It's cold, dark, and unstimulating here. You provide us with much-needed diversion. You will accept all of our invitations." And we did.

One of the invitations was to the quarters of a Veterinary Corps captain and his family. Captain Zepp greeted us at the door with an infectious grin and an even more infectious enthusiasm for Army life. He was the type who made the best out of every challenge the Army threw at him. His living room was dotted with the pelts of Arctic wolves he'd shot himself. He was an unapologetic hunter who reveled in the thrill of a successful hunt. Years later it would prove to be a fortuitous meeting.

We surveyed a couple of infantry companies of over 100 men each. We didn't find anything attributable to the Mickey Mouse boot. Therefore we had little to show for our trip. Any benefit derived would be dependent on making the most of our simply being in Alaska in the winter. Our hosts at Fort Wainwright were quick to offer assistance.

We expressed interest in surveying an indigenous population. In doing so we learned that the term "Eskimo," now preferably referred to as Inuit, is used for the coastal populations, whereas the term "Indian" is employed for people living inland. We arranged a visit to an Indian village a helicopter ride west of Fairbanks. On the appointed day we could not go; the chief's son was found frozen to death just outside his front door after a night of heavy drinking. We went three days later.

The airstrip where we landed on skis was on a raised area a quarter mile from the village. Ground transportation was provided by the village in the form of a teenaged couple in a late-model car. The driver executed a beautiful 180-degree turn on the ice by applying the brakes and steering wheel just so. The couple used head nods to indicate we should get in the back seat for the ride. Not a word was spoken as they put their noses in the air. It was as though we did not exist.

The chief told me things were good until the white man came. Then things got worse and worse until tragedies such as his son's death were commonplace. It was the Indian version of everything being better in the good old days when life was pure. I wondered if he would trade the present mode of existence for a return to the old ways: hunting without rifles; traveling without cars and snowmobiles; no doctors, hospitals, and modern medicines; and no government-built housing and welfare benefits. I didn't confront him with the issue.

The Indian village consisted of a dozen prefabricated houses with wooden siding. There was nothing individualistic about them; they were just drab-looking government issue.

The houses were sparsely furnished. Each of the three I saw had a communal atmosphere. One of the houses was used to conduct the survey. The Indians' feet were unremarkable.

On the helicopter flight back to Fort Wainwright, we could see wildlife close-up from the air. A moose was scared into a run because of the noise from the helicopter.

We had a few more days in Alaska till our flight back to San Francisco. Our surveys were completed. So we decided to hop a flight to Barrow, the settlement at the northernmost tip of Alaska. Dead Horse was the stop before Barrow. Both abut the Arctic Ocean. A half-dozen contract workers got off at Dead Horse to work on the oil rigs. They looked just like the low-level contract workers I'd seen a half-dozen years before in Southeast Asia during the Vietnam War: scruffy roustabouts who drifted from job to job but could easily find work because of the scarcity of labor.

Dead Horse was the bleakest-looking place I'd ever seen. No wonder the horse died.

At Barrow there was blinding whiteness wherever you looked. You couldn't tell where the land left off and the sea began. It was no harder to walk on water than on land. It felt almost biblical. It also reminded me of an encounter with Eskimo reserve troops during my Special Forces training at Fort Bragg. The troops were flown in from their home village on the edge of Saint Lawrence Island in the Bering Straits, some 35 miles from the Siberian mainland. The men made a subsistence living hunting sea mammals such as walruses and seals. There were no trees. When they went to sea in small hide-covered boats to hunt, they were able to find their way home despite fog and the uselessness of magnetic compasses that far north. Contrast this with how they were on a field training exercise in the Uwharrie National Forest in North Carolina. They shivered with cold despite the ambient temperature being about the freezing level instead of 50 or more degrees colder as it was on their island. They got lost in a thinned-out, leafless forest despite having compasses and maps. And they ignored any order given by anyone other than their team commander, who was also their tribal chief and the mayor of their village.

How could this be? The explanation need not be detailed. The Arctic cold is a bone-dry cold; the North Carolina cold is a wet cold. This has everything to do with the chill factor. The forest is a mystery to those who have 30 words for different types of snow to cope with and who can navigate by the stars. Wouldn't we non-Eskimos get lost in the seemingly endless, formless tracts of the Arctic winter? And, to them, we Special Forces Officer-trainees were no more than strangers in a strange land. At least they did not shoot at us.

In Barrow, when walking from building to building, I noticed that the workers didn't put up the hoods to their parkas. So as not to seem effete, I pulled my hood down. My ears became intolerably painful in 30 seconds. I ducked around the corner and replaced my hood. Better effeteness than pain. But what about the workers: Did they become cold-adapted? Animals like crows, moose, wolves, hares, and foxes certainly did, but only after millennia of evolutionary pressures. The seemingly quick adjustment of humans ran contrary to what I'd been taught. A mystery.

On the way back to Fairbanks, we re-crossed the Brooks Range that horizontally transects northern Alaska. I kept wondering what might happen if the plane developed engine trouble and we had to crash-land in the extremely rough terrain of the Brooks Range. I estimated our chances of survival at exactly zero. If the landing itself didn't kill us, surely the cold and exposure would. This was not a trip I'd care to repeat.

Before we headed back to San Francisco, we spent the evening in downtown Fairbanks. We had the opportunity to meet the former Army doctor who was the resident expert on cold injury. He in turn introduced us to the state's lieutenant governor, who happened to be visiting the restaurant-nightclub we were sitting in. It was a reminder of how small, in a population sense, our largest state really is. Everybody seems to know everybody else. This may be one of the main reasons for Alaska's appeal to some people. Others, like Walt and me, were perfectly content to return to foggy, rainy San Francisco.

Captain Zepp, the veterinarian I had met in Alaska, and I met up again some six years later when he was a member of an inspector general (IG) team that inspected Army medical facilities across the country. He greeted me as though no time had passed since our first meeting and added that he needed to tell me about something.

He recounted that he had recently visited Fort Campbell, Kentucky, where the preventive medicine chief was a physician instead of a nurse, environmental hygienist, or veterinarian like himself. This was an unusual but not a negative finding. The physician was well prepared. Even the brass on his uniform was polished. The team's next stop was Fort

Jackson, South Carolina, where the preventive medicine chief was also a physician. Again, the physician was well prepared and his brass was polished.

At the end of the first day of a two-day visit to Fort Jackson, Captain Zepp said he lay awake in bed pondering the extreme unlikelihood of two well-prepared, neatly uniformed physician chiefs in a row. At the end of the second day of inspection, he voiced his perplexity to the Fort Jackson preventive medicine chief, who said: "The answer is simple. The Fort Campbell chief and I took our preventive medicine residency training together. Our residency training director was Colonel Masters."

Case closed.

GUAM

Who hasn't been enticed by the prospect of spending a few weeks on a sun-drenched tropical island, surrounded by beautiful blue water? What if, in addition, it was an all-expenses-paid trip, and you didn't even have to pay for gas? Such was the case when, in 1975, the Army sent me to Guam, the largest island in the Southwest Pacific's Mariana chain.

It was the end of the Vietnam War. Thousands of Vietnamese refugees were streaming into Guam to be processed before being sent on to the US mainland. They had escaped by any means possible, including flimsy, leaking boats, as the South Vietnamese government collapsed when US aid and assistance were withdrawn. The refugees were housed and fed on an abandoned airstrip once used by the Japanese in World War II.

The refugees were living in field conditions: They were housed in tents, fed in soup-kitchen style, and used communal bathroom facilities. It was a setup for the spread of infectious diseases. An epidemic would be the second consecutive disaster in the lives of the refugees, especially among the most vulnerable parts of the population, the babies and the elderly.

The US Army had sent in a full medical contingent to deal with the refugees. Included was a preventive medicine unit, the Army name for a public-health contingent. At the start of the evacuation operation, the preventive medicine chief was a public health-trained doctor, a lieutenant colonel in the Medical Corps. A month into the operation, he was informed that there was a family tragedy and he was sent home. I was to be his replacement. We knew each other because we had trained together at Walter Reed several years earlier. On paper, we were very much alike.

The civilian airline flight from my home unit in San Francisco landed in Guam as the tropical sun was rising. A couple of soldiers from my new unit met me at the airport and whisked us off to a McDonald's for a 5:30 AM breakfast. Then it was off to the refugee processing camp.

There were 15 or so members of the preventive medicine unit composed mainly of public health nurses and enlisted sanitarians. Heading the sanitarians was a captain in the Medical Service Corps, a position that usually called for being the most military of the lot. After familiarization briefings, I was taken to meet the commander of the entire medical contingent, a Medical Corps colonel of long experience. We hit it off immediately.

It quickly became evident that we were entering an unofficial Phase Two of the refugee evacuation operation. Phase One included setting up the facilities, establishing procedures, and undergoing scrutiny by the media. After the first month this had become routine and the media drifted away. There was one problem with this state of affairs: Complacency would only heighten the possibility of an epidemic.

Key to preventing an epidemic would be a fully functioning sanitary component, the Army term for which was an environmental health unit, headed by Sam, its captain. From the first, Sam seemed anxious to talk to me about something. He spoke highly of my predecessor but said he was frustrated because there was a style-of-management conflict. Sam looked relieved when I told him I was more of a delegator than my predecessor.

Guam and the rest of the Marianas was a US Navy command, headed by a rear admiral, and so the Army medical group, along with the Army support group above it, had to consider this at all times. The admiral's surgeon, a naval captain, held weekly staff meetings, which my boss, the Army medical group commander, was expected to attend. I was invited to attend as well. This was the forum for airing significant concerns and getting official approval for changes in policy and practices.

From the first meeting it was obvious that the admiral's surgeon and my medical group commander were uncomfortable with one another. My commander had to defer to the admiral's surgeon because it was a Navy island. However, the colonel who was my commander was far senior to the surgeon in experience and length of service, and this was threatening. The two of us agreed on a new approach as we went around the table. He would outline a problem in such a way as to generate concern; I would follow up with the recommended means to alleviate the concern. Coming from me, a rank lower than the admiral's surgeon, the tension was greatly reduced and approval almost guaranteed.

The public health nurses were busy around the camp seeing that people got such things as medications and infant formula. The environmental health technicians were busy too, checking on sanitation. But there was a growing problem in which they were immersed. Sam, their captain, told me that there were frequent disputes between the technicians and the infantrymen, whose lot it was to clean the wooden latrines. Arguments broke out over such things as "How clean is clean?" and "Why do I, an infantryman who is trained to fight wars, have to listen to you, an odd kind of medic?" I told Sam to talk again with the infantry company commander. The company commander was reportedly as tired and dispirited as his men. Not a good sign.

I directed Sam to develop an objective set of criteria to rate the cleanliness of the latrines and put it in writing. It was to be used as a standard for the technicians and as the basis for a consolidated daily report. In addition, I suggested something he might tell the infantry company commander if complaints of tiredness persisted.

The matter of the written criteria and the report was broached at the next meeting with the admiral's surgeon and was met with strong approval. From then on I could confidently know the daily status of each of the scores of latrines should this become an issue. A summary report was submitted daily to both chains of command, line and medical.

Three days after I gave Sam his directive, he asked if I had a few moments for a progress report on the latrine issue. I could see that he was struggling to maintain a detached professional demeanor and to suppress a broad, satisfied grin. He proceeded to relate the results of his most recent meeting with the infantry company commander. Getting the usual complaints from the infantry captain that he and his men were tired, overworked, and not cut out for endless latrine duty, Sam decided to use my suggestion to bring the matter to a head and resolve it. I had suggested that he listen sympathetically to the other captain and then, in a gesture of goodwill, offer to take over command of the infantry company in addition to performing his other duties. This apparently had an electrifying effect on the other captain. All of a sudden he was energized. No more complaints about his lot in life on Guam.

A few days later I was pleasantly surprised to learn about the fate of the daily latrine report when it was submitted to the Army command group. It was not only read by the full-colonel commander, but it was the first thing he read each morning at breakfast. It was used as a management report. He now had a tool to direct and evaluate the activities of the lieutenant-colonel commander of the infantry battalion from the 25th Infantry Division, the so-called Pineapple Division from Hawaii.

The lieutenant colonel subsequently became embittered about the effects of these reports and never missed an opportunity to loudly call me "Mr. Clean" in the officers' mess. It was so childlike and inappropriate that I wondered how long such an individual would last in combat.

With public health matters now on autopilot, there was time to explore the island. Most of it was heavily forested with tropical trees such as palms. It was beautiful until you got up close. Then you noticed that virtually the entire island was heavily littered with solid waste, such as empty McDonald's wrappers. It was a complete turnoff.

Just off the beaches were coral atolls, much of it brain coral, a highly prized souvenir. Also noteworthy were the rusted remnants of steel emplacements designed to deter landing craft attempting to retake the island from the Japanese during World War II. That they ultimately failed to prevent the US from taking the island from Japan made it seem more than a bit ironic to see hordes of Japanese tourists, mostly honeymooning couples, landing at the airport and thereby re-invading the island.

When duty called again it was about some potential health problem involving preparation of food in the Army-run soup kitchens. For this I needed to coordinate with the officer in charge of logistics. The tour of the facilities and the solution to the problem were unremarkable. On the other hand, the officer, an infantry major and a graduate of West Point, certainly was remarkable. He had every conceivable badge and ribbon on his uniform. He said he had done about everything a person can do in the Army. I believed him. But I didn't believe him when he said he was resigning after 16 years of active duty. "Why?" I asked, knowing that he was only four years away from a pension. His answer: "Because I've had all the laughs." With no more meaningful challenges left to him in the Army, he wanted to enter the business world and start anew. Seen from his point of view, I was in absolute agreement. It was his time to move on.

One of the daily sights in the refugee camp was of the honey-sucker truck and its driver, a lean, weather-beaten man constantly smoking a cigarette. He worked barehanded at his job, emptying the canisters at each latrine of their contents of human waste. He placed the long hose with the metal nozzle into the "honey" and applied suction. Sometimes the nozzle became clogged with solids, a situation that he quickly rectified by removing the material with his hand. Then he would use that hand to smoke a cigarette. I was thankful that he was not my employee to supervise and that his work habits did not threaten the health of the refugees.

After two weeks of absolutely perfect, invariable weather, daily weather reports and forecasts seemed increasingly monotonous and ridiculous. I began to long for a severe weather warning, perhaps a nice typhoon blowing in from the South China Sea. Anything for a change. The island seemed smaller and more confining with each passing day. I couldn't imagine being confined to a ship or a similar island for months at a time. I was increasingly pleased that, years earlier, I had decided to drop out of Naval ROTC during my freshman year at college.

Mother Nature did not completely disappoint in terms of providing for change. She arranged for the sudden appearance of a seemingly inexhaustible supply of giant toads. Toads were everywhere. They were hideous and croaked incessantly. They insisted on crossing roads in spite of traffic. Their flattened carcasses lay in the sun and desiccated. I eagerly looked forward to getting off the island and never seeing a dried toad again.

In two more weeks the last refugee would be processed and we could go home. We were ready. Just when we thought we were nearly home free, a storm suddenly appeared. It was not a change in the weather; it was a late Friday afternoon call for my medical commander and me to report immediately to the admiral's office. I couldn't imagine what had happened.

It was my first meeting with Admiral Morrison. He was calm and even-voiced when he said he had received disturbing reports about sanitary operations at the refugee camp. There were allegations of arbitrary and unnecessarily strict sanitary inspections, of a system run amok. He said he was involved not only because the refugee evacuation was taking place within his command but also because it involved Navy personnel who were providing logistical support that included the latrines and food service.

With my commander's full backing, I responded by first giving an overview of sanitary operations and the roles of the various personnel involved. Then I homed in on the system I had Sam create and that, as a result, I could provide accurate status reports as of that very afternoon. I think he found our remarks credible because he picked up the phone and called the officers' club and asked for a certain naval captain. The officer who answered the phone was laughing and shouting at the other officer to come to the phone. When queried about who was on the phone, the question was laughingly asked, "Well, who did you say is calling?" Admiral Morrison said who it was. I envisioned the response when the message sunk in. All of a sudden it was "Yes sir! Right away, sir!" Shortly thereafter, the newly arrived naval officers were given to understand that their duties did not end on early Friday afternoon and, furthermore, there was work to be done, starting now. Even though largely *pro forma*, I still treasure the letter of commendation I received from Admiral Morrison.

Word got out concerning this calm, methodical, in-control man: He was the father of the wild rock star Jim Morrison of The Doors, who died of an overdose in Paris four years earlier. It seemed unreal.

One of the doctors assigned to the Army medical contingent was allowed to return to the US mainland a week early because he was getting married. In celebration, he threw a party at a Mexican restaurant. Each table had a pitcher of margaritas. Any other drinks were to be at the invitee's expense. Shortly after performing a more than passable guitar medley, the soon-to-be bridegroom said there would be unlimited margaritas at each table. I was among those who took him up on his generous offer. When it was time to drive back to my quarters, I was stopped at the entrance gate by the sentry, a member of the Shore Patrol, the Navy's version of the Military Police. His queries did not sit well with me, partly because I was sick of being on Guam and partly because the margaritas were having an effect. It is sobering to think that I might still be there if I had carried out what was going through my mind.

On the flight back to San Francisco, I reflected on the month on Guam. Despite the hurdles, I had a feeling of satisfaction about the assignment. My training and prior experience had paid off. Above all, there was no epidemic of life-threatening disease.

A year after the operation, designated "New Life," I began a new assignment as chief of preventive medicine at Fort Ord,

California. I bought a house in nearby Pacific Grove, a restored Victorian with stained-glass windows and a view of Monterey Bay. At the hospital were two people whom I had served with on Guam. I invited them to my house for a home tour and for reminiscing about our shared experience. Tom was a Medical Service Corps captain, an administrator; Anne was a nurse, a lieutenant colonel. Tom brought a beautifully wrapped gift for Anne, undoubtedly a token of their friendship. I was honored to be the host at this unexpected gift giving. Anne opened the card, with its effusive thanks for her friendship and support while in Guam. Then off came the gorgeous ribbon. When the large square gift box was opened, it contained scads of tissue paper wrapping the gift itself. Finally, she reached the bottom of the box where lay the gift. Anne gingerly pulled aside the last layer of tissue paper, revealing—what else?—a squashed and desiccated Guamanian toad. A perfect gift for the occasion. Tom was rolling on the floor with laughter. Anne took it well. She was heard to say: "Oh, you shouldn't have." She probably meant it literally. I was wondering: *Will I ever get Guam out of my life?* Probably not. It's been in my memory for over 35 years.

PANAMA

I thought I could get out of it based on the fact that I'd already spent 18 months in a tropical country, Vietnam, six months of which I spent investigating skin diseases among US infantrymen in wet, lowland areas. But now I was a preventive medicine resident (i.e., trainee) at the Walter Reed Army Institute of Research in Washington, DC. A mandatory part of the training was to spend a month in Panama, where the Army had a tropical medicine research laboratory. The idea was to immerse the trainees in a tropical environment so that they were less apt to experience culture shock if and when they were suddenly deployed to the tropics for military reasons.

There were four of us residents in the year 1971. We were to be in Panama at the same time. Because I'd had prior experience, I was dubbed preceptor of the group as well as being a fellow preceptee. Catch-22? Of course.

Upon arrival in Panama we spent the first week in Panama City, the capital and home of the Gorgas Memorial Laboratory, a tropical medicine research station. We were shown patients with exotic diseases at the adjacent hospital and met key staff members, some of whom were members of the world's tropical disease old-boy network. The two top researchers were Carl and Karl. When speaking of them, one was referred to as C-Carl and the other as K-Karl.

Our local liaison officer was an acquaintance, Jim, a Medical Corps major like myself. He made arrangements for us to spend most of our time in Panama in the small jungle town of Yaviza, in the eastern province that borders Colombia, the northernmost country in South America. The Darien Peninsula was the one place where the Pan-American highway, which stretches from Alaska in the North to the southern tip of Chile, had not been completed. There was a good reason for this. The Darien was extraordinarily hot, humid, rainy, undeveloped, and covered with thick jungle. It harbored hordes of mosquitoes and other disease-carrying insects, life-threatening fevers, and potentially harmful animals, such as poisonous snakes.

Transportation from Panama City was provided by US Army helicopters. I made a preliminary day-long acquaintance visit to Yaviza. It was a collection of primitive wooden shacks on a riverbank. The population was mainly composed of the descendants of blacks imported from Caribbean islands who had helped build the Panama Canal generations earlier. Nearly all the rest were Chocó Indians. One of the residents was a Chinese man who married a black woman. It was said that he knew the hourly price of gold on the world market despite his remote location. Jim had arranged for us residents to stay and take meals with a family in the nicest house in town. It had a refrigerator and running water.

Three days later I returned for a three-week stay with the other residents. The helicopter pilots, both seasoned Vietnam vets, hadn't previously been to Yaviza and couldn't find it. They circled over the monotonous triple-canopy jungle and re-consulted their maps. Finally, in frustration, they asked if I knew anything about it. I said it was on a river twice as wide as the one below us, and so it might be worthwhile to follow it downstream to see where it led. We were lucky. Yaviza was only ten minutes' flying time away.

Everybody in town seemed to know that they would have four light-skinned visitors for a couple of weeks. They were polite and receptive. Of particular note was the headman, who could schedule visits to the clinic building by the town's residents, and the young doctor, who was socially prominent and a politician as well as a physician. A few spoke halting English, which was complemented by my equally halting Spanish.

No one had told us what we were to do in the way of training activities. The only thing that was scheduled was mealtimes. The fare—morning, noon, and evening—was invariably red beans and rice. None of us developed diarrhea; the diet gave us the opposite problem.

I had decided to try to carry out a survey of the entire population for a common bacterial skin infection—pyoderma, or pus on the skin. One of the other trainees decided to survey nutritional status by taking the heights and weights of the same population. The headman was amenable to the project and arranged for manageable portions of the town's residents to show up at the clinic to be examined. We were able to survey a large proportion of the town's residents, most of whom, unsurprisingly, were children.

The town seemed to come alive as it got dark. Light was provided by a few bare bulbs powered by small generators. Out of the shadows one night emerged a bilingual US Army sergeant, Bo, a Mexican-American who went by the first syllable of his last name. He fit in easily with the citizens of Yaviza because he literally spoke their language. Bo was a medic who was sent from Panama City to monitor us and to run interference should that become necessary. He relished telling us—with a mischievous grin—of some scuttlebutt he'd heard the previous night about a plot to do something harmful to the foreigners. Us.

Prominent among the night people was a Panamanian police lieutenant, a middle-aged man who was banished to duty in Yaviza as punishment for some misdeed. According to Bo, he was heavily involved in vice and was raking off a sizable profit. Ten days after we first saw him, he suddenly vanished. A police sergeant was sent to replace him. We could only speculate as to the reasons why.

Our skin disease survey uncovered an unusual case, a large skin ulcer on the shoulder of a young logger that was eating into the deltoid muscle. We suspected it was a parasitic condition known as cutaneous leishmaniasis, which is transmitted by the bite of a sand fly. We arranged to get the diagnosis confirmed and treatment provided by the Gorgas Memorial Laboratory in Panama City. Had the skin ulcer progressed, it probably would have permanently interfered with the logger's ability to make a living. The young Panamanian doctor in Yaviza said he was unaware that such a thing existed in his community.

Travel in the area around Yaviza was mainly on the rivers, which were navigable in flat-bottomed wooden boats propelled by poles. We took a day off so we could see the area by water. It soon became apparent that getting into and out of the boats is very much an acquired skill. It made us doubly appreciative of a young Chocó man who was seen daily poling his boat in the river in front of Yaviza. He was known as the Music Man, apparently because of his renown for charming the young bare-breasted Indian women with his singing and porkpie hat. By young, I should point out that, in his society, every female became pregnant or was a mother by age 16 and therefore was too old to be among the three or four girls in the entourage of the Music Man.

We completed our surveys and took the next helicopter ride out. The obligatory exposure to the tropics of the other

preventive medicine resident trainees had achieved its purpose. Because of my previous experience in Vietnam, it was
a pointless exercise for me. However, there was some con-
solation in later months when a respected tropical medicine
journal published an article that a collaborator and I wrote on
the skin disease survey.

Eight years later, in 1979, I had another reason to visit
Panama. This time I was a full colonel and the chief of preventive medicine at the Army's Health Services Command in San
Antonio, Texas. As such, I was the top preventive medicine
consultant in the Western Hemisphere. However, that was
not the reason for my visit. Rather, it was to accompany my
Washington-based chief while he visited to help commemorate the signing of the treaty turning the Panama Canal over
to the Panamanian government. He wanted to use some of
the time in Panama to discuss with me face-to-face why I had
become involved in a flap at my headquarters in San Antonio
a few days earlier.

Taras and I spent nearly a week in Panama, primarily in
the area around the capital and the Canal Zone. We stayed
in downscale VIP quarters in the Zone. I drove the rental car
from meeting to meeting with US Army preventive medicine
and Gorgas Laboratory people as the colonel I was accompanying made his liaison visits, mostly of a symbolic nature.
Everybody we visited was aware of the US Army Medical
Department's role in making the Panama Canal possible. It was
time to reflect on the situation nearly a century earlier when a
French company gave up on its efforts to construct the canal,
in large measure because the workers fell ill or succumbed to

a variety of tropical illnesses such as malaria and yellow fever. Major Walter Reed conducted ground-breaking research on the transmission of these diseases, and General William Gorgas led the efforts to rid the area of disease-transmitting mosquitoes. This enabled an American company to finish the job the French had started.

Culture shock awaited us when we went from the Zone to surrounding areas of Panama City. Instead of uncongested roads running in straight lines, there was a seemingly impenetrable maze of narrow, crooked streets that were really no more than paved-over donkey paths dating from the days of the conquistadors.

We found that the might-makes-right approach of the conquistadors had not been lost in modern Panama. One afternoon we were driving on a clearly marked one-way street in a densely crowded part of the city. Three blocks ahead I could see a blue-painted bus headed straight for us at considerable speed. I thought surely he was going to turn off the one-lane street. But no, I was wrong. The bus kept coming without slowing. There were no side streets on which to turn off. I took the only possible alternative. I jumped the car over the curb and put the two right wheels onto the narrow sidewalk. The bus came roaring by. There were inches to spare. I almost underwent a religious conversion. Moments later, we reentered the normal chaos of Panama City and proceeded to our next destination.

Once the day's scheduled visits were dealt with, we proceeded to posh but affordable restaurants for cocktails and dinner while watching the sun set over the ocean. Then the reason for my trip came up for discussion. I explained the reasons for my actions and stated that I was unrepentant. The solution, which already had been arrived at in the Army Surgeon General's Office, was to reassign me. Problem disposed of. For the second time in my Army career, I came away from a trip to Panama with a net positive result.

A Panama Update

Now, in 2012, some 30-plus years after my second trip to Panama, several things have changed, some for the better and some for the worse.

The Panama Canal and its Zone were handed over to the Panamanian government in 1999, just as provided for in the treaty signed 20 years earlier. Fears that the Panamanians might not be capable of effectively running such a large and complex operation proved to be unfounded.

The Canal, which was completed in 1914, was built according to then-prevalent assumptions about the size of commercial and naval ships. In retrospect, the assumptions were far too limiting. The progressive increase in the size of such ships over the past century has made the Canal increasingly obsolete for a larger and larger percentage of ships, which are forced to travel thousands of extra miles if they are to navigate between the Atlantic and Pacific oceans. Stop-gap measures have been instituted, but it has become apparent that portions of the Canal will have to be re-dug in order to have the width and depth to accommodate modern shipping. Efforts to do this have begun.

Even before our trip to Yaviza in the early 1970s, considerable thought had been given to the feasibility of creating a wholly new canal. Among the sites considered, which included one in Nicaragua, was the Darien Peninsula. US Army medical research interests, coupled with those relating to a new canal, may have underlain the choice of Yaviza as a study location for us. To cut construction costs by over half, the recommended method of the excavation was to use atomic energy. Anti-nuclear political forces have precluded use of this approach.

Because of its remoteness and consequent near-absence of government control, the Darien Peninsula has become a haven for FARC guerrillas from Colombia and for drug traffickers. Indeed, the drug business in Panama flourished to the point that, in 1989, the then-dictator, Manuel Noriega, was removed from power and later convicted by the US on drug smuggling as well as other charges.

My overall impression of Panama is of a country that is defined more than most by its geography. Had it not been for a narrow isthmus between two giant continents and between two huge oceans, it would be just another banana republic, and an impoverished and even more thinly populated one at that. The narrowness of its isthmus and its strategic location remain almost its only natural resources.

SAUDI ARABIA

If you're Jewish, you're not allowed inside the Kingdom. I found this out when I was tapped to be part of a seven-man team of US Army Medical Department officers headed to Saudi Arabia in the summer of 1981. Not being Jewish was a principal criterion for selection; the others were having a specialty area and some experience in it. Therefore lieutenants were excluded. The purpose of the team was to put together a plan for the Crown Prince, the number two man in the Saudi government. He was ex officio the head of the National Guard. He wanted to create a medical establishment for his troops.

The head of the team was a lieutenant colonel, a medical administrator. The rest of the team were majors and captains, except for me, a full colonel. It bothered the team leader that, because of the difference in rank, he didn't have the same purchase on me as he had on the others. And it bothered me that not only did the Army deviate from its usual practice of having the ranking officer be the team chief, but more importantly it violated the letter and spirit of the US Constitution by excluding Jewish officers.

Preparation for the assignment consisted of reading Robert Lacey's tome, *The Kingdom,* and packing some lightweight civilian clothes. The first plane stop in the country was in Medina, a transfer point. The airport was filled with Muslim pilgrims making the *haj* to Mecca, the holiest city in Islam. I proceeded on to the capital city, Riyadh, where I joined the rest of the team in a compound on the edge of the city. It was an American enclave with all the comforts of home, except for the ambient temperature outside, which was often in excess of 120 degrees. The only saving grace was that it was a dry heat; any perspiration was instantly wicked away by the utter lack of humidity.

The team chief briefed us team members on our assignments and said that he expected to see rough drafts of our annexes to the overall plan within a week. Mine was to be on preventive medicine, my specialty. All the other medical specialties were covered by the medical administrative officers because they practiced within the confines of the hospital-based system.

At the end of the week, the other team members dutifully submitted their rough drafts for review and comment. I had not written a word. This bothered the team chief tremendously, but there was little he could do about it. For myself, I wasn't trying to be difficult; I just couldn't think of a thing to say. I wanted to get the feel of the place before I committed anything to paper.

Day trips around Riyadh revealed how oil wealth and conservative Islam created an otherworldly atmosphere. The sides of roads were littered with nearly new Mercedes and BMWs. Each had suffered a fender-bender. It was quicker and cheaper to order a new car than to repair a damaged one, however slight the damage.

Nearby, new construction was booming, all of it carried out by South Koreans expressly imported for this task. Such specialization by nationality was everywhere. Egyptians were the schoolteachers; Yemenis were the street sweepers; Americans were valued for management of complex tasks. The Saudis' work, as far as could be seen, was to lightly supervise the foreigners and to devote themselves to the practice of Islam.

The Saudis took seriously the five calls to prayer each day. As soon as the muezzin's voice was heard emanating from the mosque, everything else stopped. Restaurant staff disappeared for 45 minutes, leaving the diners stranded. Offices emptied out. Things were especially strained because it was Ramadan and the Muslims fasted from dawn till dusk.

Two events stand out because they create such sharp images of the differences between lands and cultures, between Americans and Saudis. The first was a brief tour of the National

Guard base outside Riyadh, staffed by troops recruited from the Bedouin tribes living in the desert. The mosque was the most prominent and well-kept building on the installation. But there was no running water. Consequently, the troops walked around holding plastic bottles of drinking water. An inspection of the latrine revealed dried human feces all over the floor because the toilets didn't flush. Such events showed where their priorities lay. The shortcomings, seen from an American point of view, were certainly not due to lack of money.

The other event occurred when the weekend came and we took a day trip into the desert. We went to a place that the Saudi clan used as a staging area at the turn of the twentieth century just prior to its descending on Riyadh and thereby taking over the country. We saw a small Bedouin encampment with a large black felt tent. Although their faces were heavily covered in keeping with purdah, the womenfolk fled into the tent to hide themselves from the foreign men. Outside the tent, surrounded by sand and grazing camels, was a brand-new, highly polished, black Mercedes.

On the eighth day after our arrival in Saudi, my thoughts about my assignment crystallized. I sat down and composed the preventive medicine annex in a few hours. It called for creating a preventive medicine division, with its own logistics and support system. To function effectively, preventive medicine needs to be community based, not hospital based. The team chief seemed pleased and relieved. My job was done.

I couldn't get a flight out for three more days. A sympathetic fellow colonel arranged to get me a Jeep so I could drive around town. At night, I visited the souks, seeing men holding huge wads of cash held together by rubber bands.

Nobody was concerned about thievery because the punishment was to cut off the right hand or to force the thief to flee to the desert, where a sure death from dehydration would ensue. The same fate awaited anybody who tried to steal the heavy gold jewelry displayed openly for the women to try on. Jewelry shopping for them was made especially difficult by the heavy black veils. Only the eyes could be seen.

The day before I left, I asked the team chief if he'd had a chance to review my draft of the preventive medicine annex to the plan. He said that he had. He said that it was good but that much of it was unnecessary because preventive medicine would be placed under the administrative and support structure of the hospital. To a hospital administrator, preventive medicine was just another clinic, albeit outside the hospital. I knew the true value of my trip from that moment on. Other than experiencing the otherworldliness of Saudi, my time and effort had been wasted. I was more than ready to leave.

The first leg of the trip home was a short flight from Riyadh to Bahrain, an emirate on the Persian Gulf. The plane was a medium-sized transport with 70 seats. The flight was full. I was the only man and the only foreigner. All the rest were Saudi women. Each was heavily covered in black. Even their eyes were difficult to see because of the smallness of the slits.

As we flew over the border between Saudi Arabia and Bahrain, there was a sudden change in the passengers. To a woman, each reached up and pulled off her head coverings. Now I could see what the faces holding those intriguing dark eyes looked like. They were plain and without a trace of makeup or hair styling. Perhaps there was more than one reason for the veils.

Lest there be the mistaken impression that I have something against the appearance of Arab women, I hasten to add that I had seen a number of attractive Arab women during a ten-day trip to Egypt. The only thing I can surmise is that somehow the Saudis took a wrong turn when it came to pulchritude. Maybe the oil money will make up for it. Maybe not.

Military Madness

If you were a young adult American male in the post-World War II era from the late 1940s to the early 1970s, a central fact of your life was your susceptibility to the military draft, or universal conscription as it was sometimes called. Should you be called upon to serve, you had to do it at a time and place of the US Government's choosing. You forfeited two years of your life to a form of indentured servitude where you were told what type of work you would do, what you would wear, and how you would comport yourself. You might even get killed. Attempts to avoid the draft were termed "evasion" and could be punished severely.

It was against this backdrop that I entered the US Army in July 1966. It did not take long for me to begin to appreciate—for the first time since reading the book years before—the zaniness conveyed by Joseph Heller's Catch-22. The line I had heard in an old war movie, spoken by a sergeant, echoed in my mind: "There is a right way, a wrong way, the Army way, and my way. Do it my way." Getting along in the Army, as far as I was concerned, was doing it my way without inviting the wrath of authorities whose duties were to see that things were done the Army way.

The most important lessons were imparted during the first year in the Army. The sergeant major of the medical intelligence unit I commanded advised me: "Sir, you want to keep every scrap of personnel-related paper the Army gives you. The one you need later on will be lost." Six years later, the centralized military records center in St. Louis burned to the ground a week before a sprinkler system was to be installed. Thousands of people lost the records needed to establish their eligibility for benefits and entitlements.

A little later a full-colonel administrative officer of the unit co-located with mine took a liking to me, a newly minted captain. He advised me to learn all I could about Army regulations. He said: "For every regulation there is one that contradicts it. You want to put yourself in the position of quoting the regulation that supports what you want to do." I learned to do it my way by invoking the power of the Green Machine. I became an authority on regulations some years later when I wrote an unofficial guide titled *How to Write a Regulation*. Administrative officers approached me about getting a copy for themselves, a complete role reversal.

The mid-1960s, when I entered the Army, saw the rise of a powerful antiwar movement. It was becoming apparent that our leader, President Lyndon Johnson, was hopelessly out of his element in the role of commander-in-chief during wartime. Things got crazier, to the point that I was prevented from going to work at Walter Reed because of the burning of Washington in 1968. I had come home from the war in Vietnam only to be immersed in the war in my nation's capital. It was madness. Despite this, and even though I came from an entirely nonmilitary background, I chose to stay in the Army beyond the two years of indentured servitude. It was a life-changing decision.

INTELLIGENCE?

As a second-year surgical resident at the Veterans Administration Hospital in San Francisco, I spent many weekends at the hospital waiting for patients to be admitted. To while away the time between admissions, I escaped the dreary confines of the hospital by reading Ian Fleming's James Bond novels, favorites of President Kennedy before his assassination. Little did I think I'd ever have a shot at leading the glamorous life of an intelligence agent, but I could fantasize about exotic places, dangerous missions, and femmes fatales. The only things I could be sure of in my residency were chronic sleep deprivation, seemingly endless hours assisting in the operating room, and a virtually nonexistent personal life. Not a way to live one's life to the fullest, I thought.

I had already decided to switch from general to plastic surgery, but I still had to have three years of general surgery residency training before entering the two-year plastic surgery residency. The head of plastic surgery told me that the third-year requirement was recently tacked on for purely political reasons. The first thing to be done in plastic surgery training was to "un-teach" what you had just learned in the third year. Absurd, but true.

A resident several years ahead of me had gotten constructive credit for the third year by virtue of keeping track of the operations he'd performed during his two years in the Navy. What a perfect way to kill two birds with one stone: get my military obligation out of the way and get credit for a third year of training. Despite the uncertainties, it was a temptation that was impossible to resist.

I notified the Army that I'd voluntarily join in July 1966 and flew back to Washington, DC for a few days that spring to implement my plan. A fellow resident got wind of my impending trip and recommended contacting his mother, who was the secretary to a congressman from South Carolina. She made a couple of phone calls, and the next thing I knew I had an appointment to meet the commanding general at the Walter Reed Army Hospital on the outskirts of DC. The commander, a two-star general, broke scrub in the operating room to escort me around. My plan was working, or so I thought. And how nice the Army was being to one of its future doctors, even if only for two years. It had escaped my attention, or even my understanding at that point, as to the implications of my friend's mother being the secretary to the chairman of the House Armed Services Committee, the Honorable Mendel Rivers, a staunch pro-military figure with plenty of military activities in his congressional district. He also held the military purse strings.

The honeymoon was short-lived. The following day I went to downtown DC to seek out the Army Surgeon General's personnel office to fill out paperwork. The address I had didn't correspond to anything related to the Army. It stated clearly: Main Navy Building. That was my welcome to the Washington bureaucracy. An old Washington hand wouldn't have batted an eye. It didn't have to make sense that a major component of the Army was located in the Main Navy Building or that the building itself was a rat-infested, so-called temporary building, a holdover from World War II, which ended 20 years earlier. It was simply the way things were.

I eventually found the Main Navy Building after several false starts based on, to me, the logical assumption that the Army Surgeon General's office would be located in a building labeled Army. After other false starts and after I had reached the Main Navy Building, I finally found the personnel office, a cavernous room with dozens of olive-drab desks lined up in rows. Just at the entrance was a receptionist who handed over a stack of forms that were to be completed in the hallway and returned as soon as they were completed. I dutifully complied and was especially impressed when one form was headed Assignment Preferences. How considerate of the Army.

I returned to the cavernous room only to find it almost completely deserted. It was 11:40 AM and nearly all the employees had fled their desks promptly at 11:30. The holdout was a clerk eating his bag lunch at the far end of the room. As I neared him, he stopped in mid bite of his sandwich and said loudly, "Don't show me. Let me guess." He then rattled off the name of five countries, four of which were in Western Europe. He added, "They may not be in the same order as yours, but I bet they're the same countries you entered on your assignment preferences form. Am I right?" I nodded yes. He triumphantly added: "They all say the same thing. We just send them where we want them." It was dawning on me that I was at the not-so-tender mercy of the bureaucracy.

At the end of June 1966, I left my surgery training and headed to Fort Sam Houston, home of the medics, in San Antonio, Texas. The place was packed as a result of President Lyndon Johnson's decision the year before to escalate the war in VEET-NAAM, as he pronounced it in his Texas twang. I received my orders shortly after arrival for the six-week block of basic medical officer training. I was to be a battalion surgeon in Vietnam. I had learned enough by that time to know what a nothing job that would be for me, sitting around in a tent for a year among a bunch of Americans and practicing at the level of an intern. All the interesting cases—the wounds and severe illnesses—would be flown out over my head by evacuation helicopters. And I would have no way to get to know Vietnam. I considered this an emergency.

Never volunteer. That was the standard advice from those with military experience. But I was desperate, so I went to plead with the personnel officer, a lieutenant colonel who didn't hold out much hope. He offered to contact me if anything came up in the way of alternative assignments in Vietnam. I may have exaggerated a bit when I told him of my many qualifications to do something other than being a battalion surgeon.

A month passed and still no word. Time was getting short. So I dropped in on the personnel officer, who said a requisition had just come in for a preventive medicine officer to head some kind of unit in Vietnam. None was available, so I could have the job if I wanted.

My orders were changed. I was to report to the Army Surgeon General's office in Washington to get briefed on my new assignment. It was off to the Main Navy Building again, only this time with some foreknowledge of the bureaucratic jumble.

I wended my way through the maze of offices and found the one specified in my orders. I was greeted warmly by a captain in the Medical Service Corps. After several minutes of chitchat, he said, "You know why you're here, don't you?"

So as not to admit my total ignorance, I gave a noncommittal nod of the head, to which he replied, "Just to make sure you know, you're the next commander of the medical intelligence detachment in Vietnam."

It took a few minutes for this to sink in. When it did, I began to have James Bond-type fantasies. They did not last long. Reality returned when the briefings started.

Typically, I would report to the specified officer, usually a rank or two above me, in his or her office at the designated time. After being offered the obligatory cup of coffee, the briefer would politely ask why I was there and what I wanted to know. I lamely replied that I didn't know; I thought that was the purpose of the briefings. The absence of a structured training experience became readily apparent. The briefers would tell me a version of their recently completed tours in Vietnam. No mention was made of anything having to do with medical intelligence. The closest anyone got to anything medical was when an administrative officer stated that he never had a dry fart when he was in Vietnam.

The Surgeon General's Intelligence Office liaised with sister governmental agencies, such as the Defense Intelligence Agency (DIA), the Central Intelligence Agency (CIA), and the Army's intelligence installation at Fort Holabird, Maryland, just outside of Baltimore. I went to each for briefings. The content was unimportant, but the context was revealing. Collectively, they reminded me of the cartoon caption, "Whoops, you're stepping on my cloak and dagger."

My chief recollection of the CIA headquarters at Langley, Virginia, just outside of Washington, was of stepping into a large, white, bare reception area whose walls were pierced with many holes, presumably containing a variety of sensors to monitor visitors. Another was of being followed into the men's room by my card-wearing watcher lest I collect or disseminate unauthorized intelligence while urinating.

The DIA was more of a blur, and a gray, uninteresting one at that. Getting in and out of the DIA headquarters was bureaucracy run amok. There were two sets of guards, one Army, the other civilian. The civilian guards were more economical, and that is why they were hired, but their union wouldn't let them work the night shift. The Army was called upon to fill in the gap, but the rules were that they were all or none; so soldiers were on hand 24 hours a day. Nobody was in charge of coordinating the activities of the two types of guards. It showed.

In preparing me for my visit to Fort Holabird, Jon, the captain who coordinated my briefings, said to be on the lookout for some distinctive features. "First," he said, "you'll notice the railroad track running right through the installation, thereby allowing unwanted visitors to walk in, unhampered by fences. Second, note the nondescript three-story brick building that sits just across the street from the official entrance to the installation. It looks directly on to the headquarters building, and it is rented by a Soviet spy agency. The last thing to notice is the large number of aged-looking majors of Japanese ancestry wandering about." While Jon didn't say it, this represented the institutionalized racism of the Army at the time. The Intelligence Corps was viewed as a dead-end from a careerist's point of view.

The only concrete thing I learned in three weeks of briefings was the meaning of the acronym SICR, or specialized intelligence collection request. A SICR was sent out on an ad hoc basis. Receiving one was not an everyday event. The everyday activities of an intelligence unit? I hadn't a clue.

I arrived in Saigon in September and had two weeks of overlap with my predecessor, a Medical Corps captain like myself. He had found a home for the 12-man detachment in a three-story medical facility rented from a Vietnamese doctor by the Walter Reed Army Institute of Research (WRAIR) based in Washington, DC. It was thought that the WRAIR team and the intelligence detachment would have interests in common.

My new unit belonged to an element of military intelligence called technical intelligence. The technical role was emphasized by the unit being composed of enlisted medics and two junior Medical Service Corps officers. So the members of the unit had no background or training in intelligence. We worked for the Military Assistance Command Vietnam joint intelligence staff (MACV J-2) but were assigned to the US Army Vietnam's military intelligence battalion, an entirely separate entity. It was unclear what we were supposed to do and how to do it, a situation ripe for snafus.

My immediate superior on arrival was a West Point major from the Ordnance Corps. He led me into my first battle, into an ambush of sorts. He told me to accompany him to a meeting with the one-star general in charge of MACV J-2. With no preamble, General McChristian asked me how the malaria study was coming along and when could he expect to receive a report. I had a vague recollection of some mention of a malaria study by my predecessor, but didn't know its status, and said so. I quickly learned how it felt for a captain to be dressed down by an angry general. I was sent off to obtain blood samples from enemy prisoners for malaria testing.

On delving into the malaria survey of prisoners, there seemed to be some confusion about its legitimacy. A US Navy lawyer wrote an opinion that forcibly taking blood samples for survey did not violate the Geneva Convention or the Laws of Land Warfare based on it. But of course the enemy—the North Vietnamese and Vietcong—was not a signatory to the convention. Furthermore, there was an old Vietnamese saying that one drop of blood was equivalent to one bowl of rice, thereby indicating an entirely different cultural view of the taking of blood. A preliminary visit to the POW camp at Long Binh resulted in an uprising of the prisoners that was put down by the military police guarding the camp. The malaria survey project came to a screeching halt and was never referred to again.

A couple of months went by and nothing from MACV J-2 until late one Friday afternoon. With no prior notice we were tasked to provide backup information for a briefing that McChristian was scheduled to present the following Monday to Robert McNamara, the Secretary of Defense. A senior colonel on McChristian's staff informed us that his general had already prepared the briefing; our task as subordinate unit heads was to supply backup information. In other words, conclusions first, data second. McNamara was a former Ford Corporation "whiz kid" and was reputed to devour large quantities of charts, graphs, and tables at a sitting. Woe befell the briefer who didn't have an impressive array of statistics at hand, and so they were furnished.

Management-style charts adorned the walls of the J-2 headquarters. The most arresting was the one purporting to show when the war would be won, perhaps the most important question on the minds of many Americans. On the horizontal axis was the timeline in months; on the vertical axis were two measures, as I recall, body counts and enemy infiltration. The idea was when the two lines on the vertical axis crossed, the enemy would have to give up and the war would be over. The date shown was April 1967. I expressed some skepticism of this to some of my fellow officers. A week or so later, in late fall of 1966, I received an unannounced visit from two Intelligence Corps officers, one a major and the other a captain like me. They appeared to be upset. The major made it clear that the purpose of the visit was to put me in my place. He explained that the captain had a PhD in mathematics, and even though I had a doctorate degree, mathematics trumped medicine when it came to charting prognostications concerning the war. I conceded that the captain could probably run circles around me when it came to numerical calculations, but I wondered how good were the assumptions and input data that went into the calculations. I didn't need to add that a medical degree trumped a mathematics degree when it was a matter of toeing the party line or not. The visit was not satisfying for either side.

I saw the captain from time to time at noon in the officer's mess. Whenever he saw me, he immediately headed for the other side of the room as though he might be contaminated by being seen with me. There was no acknowledgment of any kind when April 1967 came and went, and the enemy refused to lay down arms. So much for the credibility of the US Army's Intelligence Corps. As a wag once said, the value of US military intelligence was measured in terms of pounds and inches of paper reports, and not in such things as timeliness and accuracy of target locations.

For security reasons, intelligence organizations are highly compartmentalized. This has undoubted advantages in limiting the damage that moles and leakers can do, but severely limits feedback as to the effectiveness of intelligence activities. Unsurprisingly, when I requested feedback from Washington, all I got back were vaguely worded "atta boys." So I decided to go see for myself, the only problem being the distance between Saigon and Washington.

Serendipity arrived in the form of a report from an infantry division about rats being tethered around the entrances of enemy tunnels. Speculation swirled. Were they there to augment food supplies or serve as pets? Since some were dead, and plague bacteria were cultured from them, could they be in preparation for conducting a crude form of biological warfare? After all, throwing disease-ridden carcasses into enemy camps had been practiced since at least medieval days.

The way to definitively sort out whether this was a biological warfare threat or not was to provide plague cultures to the Army's infectious disease center at Fort Detrick, Maryland, an hour's drive northeast of Washington. But how to get there safely? By using the tamper-resistant bright red boxes used by our WRAIR colleagues for similar purposes. But what if something happened to the box while in transit? What about a plane crash? What if the box was broken, the plague cultures strewn around, and the media got wind of it? I presented this scenario to my superiors and suggested that having a medical officer escort the box to its destination might alleviate concern.

I was soon on my way to the US East Coast via a stopover at Elmendorf Air Force Base in Alaska. The plane was an enormous cargo transporter, this time carrying empty pallets and plague cultures. The pilot invited me into the cockpit as we flew over Western Canada and the central US at night. Out the window one could see entire regions of the two countries. I had a sense of otherworldliness.

The authorities at Ford Detrick were underwhelmed by the plague cultures. There was nothing special about them from a biological warfare point of view. I didn't fault them. If I had been asked, for example, by the colonel who signed my orders, whether in my judgment a trip by a professional escort was in order, I would've said no. But I was never asked for my judgment, and made use of that situation in getting back to Washington.

The week in Washington was a pleasant interlude, but a dry run in terms of finding out whether my unit's reports were having any impact on the intelligence system. It was like shadowboxing; there is an image of activity, but little substance. It was time to face facts and stop trying to improve the system. Just return to Vietnam, put in my time, and return to the world, as the expression went.

As the year wore on, I realized that I had lost any desire to return to surgery training. The chance co-location with the WRAIR Special Forces team suggested another professional route. I could try an assignment with the team. If it worked out, I could follow up with a preventive medicine residency in the Army and become a board-certified specialist. This is exactly what I did. It worked well.

Looking back at the year as an intelligence agent of sorts, I have mixed emotions but no regrets. It never surprises me when there are repeated reports of US intelligence failures.

The superb Special Forces training, followed by the equally superb WRAIR Global Medicine course, were extraordinary experiences. These opportunities would not have come were it not for being an ersatz James Bond.

GOING AIRBORNE

Toward the end of my yearlong tour of duty in Vietnam as an "obligated volunteer" (meaning I would be drafted if I did not sign up voluntarily), I made two life-changing decisions: I would stay in the Army beyond the period required, and I volunteered to join the elite US Army Special Forces. My motives were several: I wanted to escape returning to the drudgery of a surgical residency; I felt like trying a stint in something related to public health before considering switching specialties from surgery to preventive medicine; and I had seen how well trained, supported, and led were the members of the Special Forces component of the Walter Reed Army Institute of Research team in Vietnam. Joining the Special Forces—the Green Berets—required that you pass a physical examination and become "jump qualified" before being allowed to begin Special Forces training. To become jump qualified, it was necessary to complete a three-week block of parachute training at Fort Benning, Georgia. The physical was a breeze; the parachute training was something else.

I should point out that I have always been afraid—no, terrified—of heights, especially precipitous drop-offs of hundreds of feet. The thought of jumping out of an airplane into the void, with only a fallible parachute between me and utter oblivion, would ordinarily have deterred me altogether. But I was not, for the reason that the parachuting was not an end in itself; it was the means to a much more important goal—becoming a Green Beret. It also was a first lesson in coping with fear: have an overriding goal.

I arrived in Fort Benning in October, a perfect time of year because it was neither too hot nor too cold. I drove up the long, beautifully landscaped entrance drive to the headquarters and signed in. Shortly thereafter, I found my new home for the next three weeks, a wooden World War II-era temporary structure that was so termite ridden and otherwise derelict that it was scheduled for demolition just after our group completed training. These were junior officer quarters, which meant one person per room. The quarters for enlisted trainees were similar, but instead there were multiple men per room. I didn't care about the quarters, just the training. Having acquired our quarters, the next thing was to have our heads shaved—a ritual that was repeated weekly.

We awoke before sunrise (oh dark 30 in military lingo) to begin training. We formed up willy-nilly. I had never been in a formation like that before, so I just placed myself fourth man back on the left column of the formation. Soon a sergeant stood at the front facing the formation and began barking commands. I didn't understand a word, so I just copied what the man in front of me did. It worked. After calisthenics, we went to the mess for breakfast and then on to the start of the first week of training.

After the first full day of training, a sergeant took the officers aside and said: "There is no dropping out. You volunteered. We discourage the enlisted from quitting, but allow it. But you men are officers. You do not quit. Period."

The entire first week was spent in learning how to fall from a two-foot-high step into a sandpit. A no-brainer, right? Wrong. There was virtue in becoming accustomed to doing things by rote. A hard parachute landing could be ameliorated by hitting the ground and falling with proper technique, letting the force be progressively taken up by the feet, calves, thighs, buttocks, and the side of the back. I asked one of the training sergeants, or cadre as they were known, why the caution about this two-foot jump into a sandpit. He replied that it was surprising how many fit young man sprained or broke their ankles because they did not follow proper technique.

The second week started the focus on the jump itself. For this there was a repeated jump out of a 34-foot tower, following which the trainee would slide down a wire into a sandpit. Then he would proceed to a line of men waiting to be critiqued about how well or how poorly he had executed the jump from the tower.

The sergeant who did the critiquing was right out of central casting. Sergeant First Class De La Garza was a hard-bitten career infantryman who looked like he had seen it all. He had a prominent Dick Tracy scar on his left cheek. His demeanor was that of an intense, hardened professional. He radiated confidence and experience, and had the undivided attention of those whom he critiqued. They would take their turn to stand at parade rest in front of his eight-foot-high seat, heads tilted far back while they listened to the critique. He would look up from his notepad, then down at the trainee with a scowl, pause, and suddenly bark his critique, which usually was anything but complimentary. The 19-year-old privates seemed petrified. They clearly respected and believed in De La Garza. It was pure theater.

Discipline was strict. At the slightest infraction, such as not sitting up straight or talking while waiting for a critique, one of the cadre would shout, "Down for ten," meaning get down on the ground and perform ten push-ups. If an officer committed the infraction, the word "sir" would be inserted after the command, as in "Down for ten, *sir*." The word "sir" would be spoken with a sneering tone of voice as though talking to a disrespected subordinate, which in fact the officer was during the period of his parachute training.

During the first two weeks, we had physical and didactic training as well. We ran in formation for two miles a day. The pace left a number of us breathing so hard that it seemed impossible to belt out the jodies—marching songs—as we were supposed to do. The cadre running beside us, usually backward, yelled every time they caught us not singing at the top of our lungs. No letup: That was the lesson.

The didactic training was about what to do inside the aircraft just before the jump, and then what to do after exiting it. Because the Army had been doing this training for so many years, the training had been boiled down to a fixed set of procedures. In the aircraft, the trooper followed the nine jump commands. After exiting, it was the five points of performance. Although I've always had a notoriously faulty memory, I can still recall the commands and points over 40 years later. Also in my memory is what to do if one comes down onto trees, power lines, or water.

Before proceeding to jump week, I ought to mention a painful lesson learned after a sergeant told us: "Gentlemens (sic), make sure that, when you are putting on your harness, to adjust your groins." I did a perfunctory job of adjusting the straps of my harness before my first jump out of the 34-foot tower. One of the straps went under my testicles instead of beside them. When I jumped, my full weight hit the sensitive part of my "groins." I never made that mistake again.

Finally, it was the third week—jump week. The class, if it can be called that, still had hundreds of men—perhaps 500—but substantial numbers had quit or were forced out by injury. Three of the five doctors who started had dropped out, allegedly because of physical injuries. Of the two remaining doctors, I was the one selected to wear the white helmet, meaning that I would be the first to jump after the "wind dummy," an experienced jumper whose job it was to see if it was too windy for the trainees to jump.

Why go first? Answer: To scarf up the trainees who got injured by hitting the skin of the aircraft when exiting, or by hitting the ground too hard or with improper technique. But when I asked who would scarf me up if I was the one who got injured, I was told, "Nobody. That's why you get jump pay, sir."

The first jump out of an airplane was a transformational experience. It had a finality about it—no going back if something went wrong. It was commitment in purest form. One had to concentrate on the task, the mission, and push personal concerns into the background.

Five jumps are required to become jump qualified and to receive the coveted jump wings, a silver-colored badge. To my surprise, the second jump was more frightening than the first. The first jump is into the unknown, but the second is just the reverse—you *know* what it is like to have only a flimsy piece of cloth keeping you from crashing to earth hundreds of feet below. Something else was distinctive about the second jump: I scarfed up the other doctor, who had broken his leg on landing. He pleaded to continue training to the finish just a couple of days away. No luck—he was sent to the hospital. He would have to repeat the entire block of training at a later date if he still wanted to earn the parachute badge.

The white helmet's purpose was to distinguish the wearer from hundreds of other trainees and thereby to allow a sergeant in a Jeep to drive the wearer around the field to evaluate the trainees who got injured during the jump. This precluded the wearer from leaving the drop zone just after he had landed, but had the compensating advantage of not having to carry one's parachute across a very large field for turn-in. It was a deal, even though it required staying while multiple plane loads of troopers jumped.

Mostly due to favorable weather conditions, the fifth and final training jump was scheduled for Wednesday instead of Thursday or Friday. It went off without a hitch. The mood of the trainees was one of elation. They had survived the training and emerged from it as proud airborne troopers. They did not walk across the field to turn in their parachutes; they ran. The beer would flow freely that night.

There was one exception to this picture: the wearer of the white helmet. Me. I was of course delighted that I had successfully completed airborne training, but I—an old man of 30—walked slowly off the field after getting out of the Jeep. A young black private came running up behind me, his face radiating pride in his accomplishment, shouting: "C'mon, doctah, youze airbohne *now*." I knew at that moment that, as fellow airborne soldiers, he would take care of me in a combat situation, and likewise I would take care of him. We were brothers under the skin.

ROLE PLAY

Unlike most other career US Army officers, doctors are not encouraged to spend part of their careers attending the Command and General Staff College. I decided to do it anyway because it might come in handy should there be a major war. Instead of the year-long course at Fort Leavenworth, Kansas, I elected the three-year night school option at Fort Ord, California, my duty station from 1976 to 1979.

Part of the schooling was a two-week summer camp at the University of Nevada campus in Reno. The curriculum was strictly focused on the knowledge and skills required of a large-unit commander and the staff officers who aided such commanders. In so-called table-top exercises, mock battles between US and aggressor (read Soviet) forces were fought with students acting as commanding or staff officers for units as large as divisions or corps, or sometimes even whole armies. For a captain or a major to be acting as an officer half a dozen ranks higher was, to say the least, a heady experience. Like my fellow students, I felt it was enormously illuminating to see what it was like to view the situation from a higher vantage point. The power of role play was self-evident.

I retired from the Army without having an opportunity to utilize any of the things I learned in Command and General Staff College. In my post-Army job I was the director of a city-county health department, seemingly unrelated to anything military. There appeared to be no transferable skills.

As part of my health director job in Tacoma, I joined an organization called the National Association of County Health Officials, or NACHO for short. Before long, I was a member of the board and attended the annual meetings in Chicago. One year, the chair asked board members to participate in coming up with educational sessions appropriate for county health directors. We were left to our own devices as to the course topic and content. My two years as a civilian health director had impressed me with how much of the job was political and how little had anything to do with the technical and professional skills acquired from public health training. Judging from what I had seen and experienced, we in public health were not very good at politics and public relations. I was determined to find out if this was generally true and to see what could be done about it.

The invitation to come up with an educational offering was the opening I was looking for. It was an opportunity for health directors to see how others, in county government and beyond, saw them. Role play seemed to be the appropriate vehicle.

At the meeting the following year, approximately 40 directors showed up for the educational session. An hour was allotted to each presenter. I was eager to see how my session would be received.

When the time came I told the group that we were going to simulate a county council meeting in Any County, USA. I would serve as chairman and would appoint members of the group to serve as fellow council members and directors of various agencies in county government. Heads of major components of health departments, such as public health nursing and environmental health, would be represented as well. I modeled things pretty much as I knew them from my home turf, Pierce County, Washington.

Besides myself as chairman, who was a centrist politically, there was a liberal who routinely championed social causes and a conservative who was a strict law-and-order type. All of us were elected officials in the county government with interests far beyond public health. Next in line were the heads of various county departments: public works, planning, parks, and social services. Last were the health department staff heads.

I appointed the role players at random from the assembled group of health directors. One, an older man, said he could not accept the appointment as the conservative council member because it would bother his conscience too much. I said these were only temporary roles, not permanent conversions of conviction. There were a couple of others who expressed similar feelings. They were adamant. They also said they had to strongly advocate for health care for the poor despite the absence of a mandate (and funding) for the health department to do so.

The rest of the group responded robustly. Nobody was surprised when the director of public works got a huge budget increase for the extension and repair of the county road system, but the health department was told, "We are sorry, but there is no money to fund public health programs such as outreach and AIDS prevention. Try again next year." Those with acting skills relished the role of the conservative council member and mercilessly slammed the health director for advocating a needle-exchange program to interrupt the transmission of AIDS. They all seemed to get the message that the health department was the weak sister in county government. In a world where there was cutthroat competition for funds, the willingness of public health people to be treated as second-class citizens had a predictable outcome.

As one of the real-life health board chairs and mayor of Tacoma once told me in an unguarded moment: "All you guys get is the crumbs off the table." He was not being deliberately harsh; he was simply explaining the facts of life. The role play drove this point home to the participants. It cast away illusions that such things as the purported lack of money were just temporary phenomena.

At the end of the session, I was approached by a young woman who asked for a word with me. Although we were both medical doctors and county health directors, we were opposite in other respects: She was black; I'm white. She was young; I was well into middle age. She went to Harvard for medical training; I went to the University of California. She worked in the Southeast (Alabama); I was from the Pacific Northwest (Washington State). From this, you might have expected that our life and work experiences would be quite different from one another. True?

I said of course she could have a word with me. She then asked me if I had ever been in her county in Alabama. I said, "Not knowingly." Then the punch line came: "What you presented in the role play was exactly how it is in council meetings in my county." It was the best feedback I have ever received. It was recognition that we were all in the same boat. The time had come to get out of our technical comfort zones and become much more effective in funding and development of political influence.

As the next year rolled around, the NACHO chair requested new educational sessions. There was to be just one repeat: role play.

THE COMMAND

It sounded impressive, rolling off the tongue in an authoritative manner. It was the brainchild and hatchling of one of the most forceful and influential of the generals in the Army Medical Department during the 20th century. It was the US Army Health Services Command, first commanded by its creator, Major General Spurgeon Neel, in 1973.

Its *raison d'être*, so it was said, was to allow the Army Surgeon General's Office in Washington, DC "to focus more on staff and technical supervisory duties," leaving most of the rest—the majority of the Army Medical Department—in the hands of the Health Services Command, or HSC as it was commonly known. A skeptic might say that two-star General Neel's preference was to be a top-level commander rather than a staff officer, and the creation of HSC was a power grab on his part. Reinforcing this notion was the fact that it reported directly to the Army Chief of Staff, bypassing such inconveniences as going through three-star generals.

As the chief of preventive medicine at Fort Ord, California, in the late 1970s, I had been a member of the Health Services Command without giving it a second thought. Anything of consequence was passed down directly from the Surgeon General's Office in Washington, as reflected in the phone call I got in early 1979. The chief of preventive medicine at HSC headquarters was retiring and I was to be his replacement. The caller, Taras, a fellow colonel who was the head of the

Surgeon General's preventive medicine section, claimed it was a significant advancement and a golden opportunity. I knew better, but was in no position to refuse the assignment.

San Antonio, Texas, did not beckon me as it had many other members of the Army Medical Department, particularly those who were approaching retirement and wanted a cushy job where they could enjoy the amenities of the Sunbelt, like near year-round golf. I had been to Fort Sam Houston in San Antonio for temporary duty assignments three times in the past, and knew firsthand that, for people like me, once you had been to the Alamo and the nearby River Walk, you had seen and done what there was to see and do in San Antonio.

The HSC headquarters occupied a three-story office building in medical row at Fort Sam Houston, home of the medics. Despite the rhetoric about leaving the specialized staff functions to the Surgeon General's office in Washington, it duplicated them. It simply added another layer to the bureaucracy. In doing so, it did little more than put a constriction on the flow of information between Washington and the rest of the country. Yet a number of the officers at HSC headquarters, especially the senior colonels, mouthed the term "The Command" in blustery yet almost reverential tones. It struck me as pure puffery.

Months went by with nothing that I found meaningful. I was fortunate enough to have an excellent staff of a dozen officers and civilians, which made things more bearable. I was struck by how little communication existed between the various offices in the building and with the commander's office. For an organization that was supposed to be adding value by clarifying directives from Washington and supervising Army medical centers and hospitals across the country, it seemed to be passive and almost uninvolved.

Then, in late 1979, I got an unexpected phone call. It was a harbinger of things to come. The caller was a Medical Service Corps administrator who had a staff job in the Army Surgeon General's Office in Washington. The major was a friendly acquaintance from ten years previously when he and I were members of the Special Forces, whose elite membership promoted a sense of camaraderie. He called me because of something he had just learned by virtue of sitting in on a planning session. He said he wanted to give me a heads-up, a warning that I was to be named the Army doctor to assist in a Central Intelligence Agency scheme in Southeast Asia. According to the caller, there had been reports from northeast Thailand of skin ulcers resulting from drops of poison falling from trees. The CIA interest was apparently to confirm or deny these reports and especially to be able to counter any Cold War propaganda that the Americans were doing something dastardly to civilians in Asia.

It did not come as a surprise that my name had been mentioned in connection with questions about skin problems in Southeast Asia. I had researched the causes of skin diseases among US Army troops in Vietnam and had written a published monograph in 1977, *Skin Diseases in Vietnam, 1965–72*, under the auspices of the Army Surgeon General. However, this was done from the standpoint of finding ways to prevent common, easy-to-diagnose skin problems that occurred in epidemic proportions in troops. It did not involve diagnosing previously undiagnosed skin problems in native populations and judging whether or not they were of toxic origin. The former calls for an epidemiologist, which I was, and the latter a dermatologist, of which the Army had a number at its disposal.

Over the next few days, I thought about the phone call and how I might respond if anything came of the planning session. The first thing that came to mind was that the CIA scheme seemed harebrained. I wanted no part of it, especially because of my low opinion of US intelligence agencies resulting from my first assignment in the Army as the head of medical intelligence in Vietnam. And I wondered what kind of involvement was envisioned for me: participation in planning a mission or throwing me into the breach as the US "expert" on skin diseases in Southeast Asian conditions.

Ironically, I had just finished giving a talk on skin diseases among troops in Vietnam to dermatology residents at the nearby Army hospital when the message from Washington came in to the command's headquarters. As I entered the building where my office was located, I heard a booming voice nearby say, "There you are. Come to my office immediately." It was the voice of the deputy commander of the Health Services Command, a fellow Medical Corps colonel. It was brusque, officious, and thoroughly condescending in tone, as though I were some kind of a truant. It immediately deepened my dislike of The Command, in my view a perfect example of the proliferation of unnecessary intermediate higher headquarters in armies across the world.

Once in the colonel's office, he informed me that a classified message had just come in from headquarters in Washington saying I was to be placed on orders immediately for a special assignment in Southeast Asia. I told him I was fully aware that something like that was afoot, had had a chance to think it over carefully, and did not think it was a good idea to blindly follow these orders. He expressed no interest in finding out why I'd take such an apparently provocative position and said he was simply following orders. I made it unequivocally clear that I had no intention of following them as such.

At this impasse, the colonel took me upstairs to meet with the commander, a two-star medical general. We had met several months before but had no other dealings. I described what had transpired in the deputy commander's office and reiterated my opposition to the orders. The general listened impassively and said the orders were what they were. I had had enough. I then said I fully realized the implications of refusing to follow a direct order and was prepared to tender my commission forthwith. I added that I was greatly dissatisfied with my assignment to the headquarters and had never wanted it. The meeting broke up shortly thereafter.

The preceding events took place on a Friday. On Monday morning I received a phone call from Taras, the chief of preventive medicine in the Army Surgeon General's Office in Washington. He had been my boss in a previous assignment and so we were well acquainted. He asked what in the world had happened. He explained that, on the previous Friday night, the three-star Army Surgeon General and the two-star commander of the Health Services Command had spent an hour and a half on the phone discussing a certain disgruntled medical officer. The upshot was to air the matter further during a trip to Panama to commemorate the treaty handing over the Canal Zone from the United States to the government of Panama. I gladly accepted the orders to accompany my Washington chief.

There were several dynamics at work. Taras was instrumental in getting me assigned to HSC headquarters in San Antonio because he thought I could strengthen the preventive medicine presence there. The general of The Command was quietly concerned about rapid staff turnover resulting from officers taking retirement or assignment changes as soon as they could. This was seen as an undercurrent of dissatisfaction with their jobs. And then there was the issue of the CIA.

My actions on "Black Friday" scotched all this. I was unrepentant. I told Taras why I had done what I did. I said I would do it again if confronted with the same set of circumstances. I told him that, in my opinion, the HSC job was meaningless. I said there was a reason why a wag had described HSC headquarters as a two-week delay in mail between DA and the field. DA, the Department of the Army in Washington, made the rules and assignments, and sent them out to the field, meaning every post, camp, and station. The Command was not to change a thing, but merely to add an endorsement that said, "Yours for information and appropriate action." What else?

Taras, whose Eastern European upbringing made him seem hyper cautious by American standards, gradually let it be known what was to become of me and the issues surrounding. I was to be reassigned from "The Command" as soon as practicable. I was no longer to be put on orders to go to Southeast Asia; an Army dermatologist was to be sent instead. And I was encouraged to not make an issue of how undesirable was the job at HSC headquarters.

Several weeks after returning to San Antonio, I heard through the grapevine that the senior dermatologist at the nearby Army medical center went to Southeast Asia, and not much became of the CIA caper. The dermatologist's wife was killed in a car crash on the way home from taking him to the airport, apparently because she swerved to avoid hitting a deer and instead hit a tree. Blindly following the orders to participate in the CIA caper had done damage to everyone touched by it, with no apparent gain.

Meanwhile, the hierarchy of "The Command" made it clear that I was to be treated like an organizational leper during my last couple of months there. I was taken off orders to go to Israel as part of an HSC delegation. And my role as part of an Inspector General team was reduced from going on the road to various medical facilities to going to the military medical training school next door.

A couple of months after being reassigned to the Army medical center in San Antonio, I unexpectedly saw a familiar face as I was leaving my building. It was Gary, the commanding general of the US Army Research and Development Command, who was visiting Fort Sam Houston on a business trip. We exchanged greetings and he then launched into a profuse apology for what had happened vis-à-vis the CIA caper. He explained by saying he had been called into a planning session and mentioned my name as knowledgeable about how to offer assistance to the CIA. He said he had stressed that I be brought into planning, but matters had gotten out of his control. I found his account credible. I visualized how some operations officer in the Army Surgeon General's Office thought he could make life simpler by the expedient of deeming me the "expert" and not immersing himself in what he regarded as technical details. Wrong move.

In 1994, 21 years after the birth of The Command and 15 years after my abortive assignment there, HSC got axed. Its functions, whatever they may have been, were merged back into the Army Surgeon General's Office in Washington. Things had gone full circle with nothing to show for the expenditure of resources. The end result reminds me of Shelley's poem, *Ozymandias*:

> I met a traveller from an antique land
> Who said: Two vast and trunkless legs of stone
> Stand in the desert. Near them, on the sand,
> Half sunk, a shattered visage lies, whose frown,
> And wrinkled lip, and sneer of cold command,
> Tell that its sculptor well those passions read
> Which yet survive, stamped on these lifeless things,
> The hand that mocked them and the heart that fed:
> And on the pedestal these words appear:
> "My name is Ozymandias, king of kings:
> Look on my works, ye Mighty, and despair!"
> Nothing beside remains. Round the decay
> Of that colossal wreck, boundless and bare
> The lone and level sands stretch far away.

THE PROFESSOR

Looking at his origins, you would give him less than a million-to-one chance of becoming a full professor in a medical school. There, every faculty member was expected to have at least one doctoral degree, MD or PhD, if not both. He had neither. In fact, he didn't even have a bachelor's degree, just certification that he was a medical laboratory technician.

Damon was one of non-identical twin brothers born in Southampton, England, in 1929. His family was working-class, meaning, among other things, that you were expected to know your place and to speak with an accent that revealed your origins. According to Damon, his father, who routinely came home drunk and belligerent, tried to prepare his sons for life by teaching them how to pilfer and steal.

After the World War II years, during which most people's chief objective was to survive the German bombing raids, Damon completed the English version of high school and enlisted in the Royal Air Force. He was sent to Palestine as a lab tech. He spent his off-hours volunteering medical services to the constant influx of Arab refugees. By his own admission, he was not a model RAF enlistee, but he learned a lot from helping the Palestinian refugees.

At the end of his enlistment, an aunt noted his aptitude for the scientific part of things medical. She encouraged him to attend the highly reputed laboratory technician training at Southampton Hospital. He got his certificate, took a job in a hospital, and married one of his fellow lab techs. It didn't take long for him to realize that advancement opportunities were severely limited in postwar Britain, and that he would have to wait for the death or retirement of whomever was ahead of him before he could move a step up on the career ladder. So he decided to emigrate to the United States.

His first employment in the US was as a hospital laboratory technician in western Massachusetts. He soon ran across endemic corruption and wanted to leave. But where to go?

At that time, 1956, a dermatologist who had been on the staff of E. R. Squibb & Sons, Inc., a major pharmaceutical firm in New Jersey, was persuaded to move to Florida to become the first professor and chairman of the Department of Dermatology of the newly instituted University of Miami School of Medicine. Dr. Harvey Blank's mandate was not only to head a teaching program for residents and medical students but also to foster research into the causes and treatments for skin diseases. For this, he needed the assistance of a well-trained and experienced laboratory technician. The word went out, Damon responded, and he was selected for the job in Florida.

Grants were the main source of funding for medical research. One potential source of grant monies was the US Army Medical Research and Development Command. Damon became not only the lab tech but also a co-investigator of an Army-sponsored research project looking into the effects on skin of a Transportation Corps exercise in the hot, humid jungles of Panama. Operation Swamp Fox, in 1961, revealed an urgent need to develop methods for bringing sophisticated laboratory tests into the field under the most difficult conditions.

It would be seven more years before I met Damon and developed professional and personal bonds that remain to this day. During this interval he authored or co-authored 30 journal articles, co-wrote a manual on recognizing and identifying dermatophytes (ringworm fungi), developed a new type of culture medium for growing and identifying disease-producing fungi, taught dermatology residents, and developed an international reputation for his work on the microbiology of the skin.

That he was not an unaspiring laboratory technician was clearly revealed when he came up for promotion. He was offered a more senior position as a technician, an offer that he refused. He held out for being placed on the academic track and was promoted to assistant professor. Damon initially encountered considerable resistance when he insisted on doing something so unorthodox, but reason held sway. He was deserving of the promotion because he had educated and otherwise proved himself to the point that he was the peer of any other faculty member.

Damon's penchant for a touch of irreverence in the face of the most sobersided science was revealed early on in his manual on the recognition and identification of dermatophytes (meaning, literally, plants on skin). Immediately after introducing a section titled "The Perfect Ascigerous State," which has to do with the sex life of fungi, he inserted a bit of whimsy:

"A pinch of dirt, a wisp of hair,
and thou beside me in the petri dish!"

He also fathered two girls, acted in locally produced plays, bought a weekend retreat in the Everglades, and rid himself of any trace of his working-class accent, substituting instead a cultivated, urbane manner of speaking.

Along with his department chairman and another dermatology professor, he made a consultant visit to Vietnam in 1967 to look into skin disease problems in American troops. They found that many infantrymen suffered from a severe form of ringworm infection, something they were well qualified to investigate.

Any investigations would be greatly facilitated by having military investigators in Vietnam dedicated to skin diseases. There happened to be a unit of Special Forces-trained doctors and medics at the Walter Reed Army Institute of Research (WRAIR) in Washington, DC, that might be amenable to providing manpower for such a task. A visit by the unit's leader to Miami in 1968 ended with an agreement that the Army would provide a team of three.

The unit's mission was to provide Field Epidemiologic Survey Team (FEST) assistance to investigations that required an ability to work effectively in a combat environment. They required additional training specific to the task at hand, such as epidemic skin diseases. Backup laboratory support and technical guidance would ordinarily be provided by the WRAIR; however, the Institute did not have an element dedicated to skin diseases. But the Department of Dermatology at the University of Miami—in the form of Assistant Professor Damon Tarpin—did have the requisite capability. Damon had prior experience in conducting field studies among troops; he developed techniques for performing microbiological studies under field conditions; and he had an almost ideal training site close at hand, the area around his retreat in the Everglades.

In July 1968 I was informed by the head of WRAIR's Special Forces unit that I had been selected to be the officer assigned to head the three-man FEST team dedicated to skin diseases. Of the officers available for assignment, I was the only one to have had a previous tour in Vietnam. This apparently weighed heavily in the selection process because the Army wanted somebody whose prior experience could enable him to hit the ground running.

In August of 1968 the two sergeants and I met in Damon's laboratory in Miami to begin our mission training. Damon and I complemented each other: I had the academic degrees; he had detailed knowledge of dermatology and microbiology. He had research experience; I had none. I had the entrée provided by virtue of being a military officer; he had to work from the periphery of the system because he was a civilian. He had published research papers, and I was new to the process.

The two sergeants complemented each other as well. One was an experienced laboratory technician; the other had been a frontline infantryman who decided to become a medic in midcareer. Both skill sets would be needed for the mission in Vietnam.

In the two months before going to Vietnam, we were occupied with training by Damon and his associates. Part of the training took place in the Everglades, a more detailed account of which is contained in the vignette, "The Everglades." Another part was participating in skin disease surveys of US Army Ranger trainees in environments ranging from mountains to coastal swamps. It was here where Damon's knack for picking up on military lingo and adapting himself to military scheduling realities became apparent.

In early October 1968 Damon and I found ourselves in a US Army headquarters north of Saigon. We were greeted warmly by the medical general, who promptly arranged for a laboratory facility dedicated to our use in the US Ninth Infantry Division's base in the Mekong Delta. Damon was designated a VIP with a protocol level equivalent to that of a full colonel.

Two days later we were at the headquarters of the Ninth Division. We were assigned to VIP quarters and met with the two-star general who commanded the division of 18,000 soldiers. Damon quickly won the general's support for conducting medical studies of selected units in the division. After supper in the officers' mess, it was off to our shared quarters for a well-deserved night's rest.

We discussed the day's events and plans for tomorrow as we drifted off to sleep. Around midnight we were awakened by a terrific noise. The ground was shaking. Despite bare visibility I could see Damon leap out of bed, do a half somersault, yell "Incoming!" and duck under his bed. Apparently he hadn't noticed that our quarters were sited in the midst of a 155 mm artillery battery and we were simply experiencing the nightly outgoing "harassment and interdiction" fire. He couldn't suppress an embarrassed grin when he emerged from under the bed.

We returned to the Walter Reed team headquarters in Saigon to gather supplies and mail. Then it was back to the Delta in our Jeep. Damon sat in back. Instead of putting his flak jacket on so that it would protect his chest from grenade fragments, he sat on it. When asked why, he replied, "I'm merely protecting my most viable parts in case there is an explosion under the Jeep."

We had to wait for a couple of hours alongside the road because the enemy had blown the bridge ahead and only a ferryboat could get us to the other side. Damon started taking pictures of the children who flocked around to try to sell us soft drinks and trinkets. Those who had their pictures taken demanded payment for the privilege. After a frantic search in each of his pockets, Damon took out a wad of piasters and peeled off bills from the top for the children. Until we stopped him, he was handing out notes worth the equivalent of US$20 when those worth a dollar would have been more than sufficient. The sergeants and I were becoming increasingly aware that, in Damon, we had the quintessential absent-minded professor.

When Damon returned to the US, we communicated by means of cassette tapes, then a technological advance. He was pleased with the results of our surveys of troop units. In a tape received just before Christmas, he didn't mention anything about season's greetings. Instead, in the event of an enemy mortar attack, he expected us to do the right thing and use our bodies to shield the notebooks containing our research data. It was an eye-opening lesson in research priorities.

When six months of data collection were up, I returned to the US and joined Damon in presenting our results in lectures and publications. He cautioned me to be especially careful about color slides illustrating our talks. When there were multiple presenters, many of them distinguished professors, it was his experience on multiple occasions that key slides would be missing by the end of the session. That this was more than accidental was revealed when, at some time in the future, the self-same slides would be shown by a presenter who had shared the podium with Damon in the past. Moreover, there was no hint of attribution, but instead the illustration was presented as though it were the presenter's own.

After the Vietnam project was completed and the results published, it would have been expected that our paths would diverge. But, in 1971, when I was a resident in preventive medicine at the WRAIR in Washington, I got a phone call from Damon in Miami. He asked if I would like to join him in conducting research in Colombia, South America. He had a colleague there who could provide key contacts in the medical community and a little laboratory space. His idea was to perform surveys of impetigo, a bacterial skin infection, at different altitudes in that mountainous country to see what effect elevation might have. I was all for it.

The following month we were in Colombia and conducted the study among children in orphanages and in Colombian Army units. The research report was well received. Damon returned to Colombia on at least five occasions to conduct further studies in the Army. In all these studies Damon used the Field Epidemiologic Survey Team concept that we had used in Vietnam. Eventually, scores of young adults—doctors, nurses, scientists, medical students, and others—were trained and led by Damon as he conducted studies in various Third World countries. It was a life-changing experience for many. They had had the privilege of being guided by a master mentor.

In 2000 Damon had reached the age of retirement from the medical school. It was time to look back on his accomplishments. He had become a full professor in two departments: Dermatology, and Epidemiology and International Health and an associate professor in Microbiology. His professional publications numbered over 150, in some 20 of which the two of us shared authorship. He had an international reputation for expertise in skin microbiology and for his ability to conduct research in Third World populations.

In celebration of his retirement, the faculty sponsored an afternoon dedicated to testimonials about Damon. At times it turned into something akin to a celebrity roast. I was unable to attend because I was on the opposite coast. But, while wearing a Green Beret, I recorded on a CD some prepared remarks I sent to Miami for use in the ceremony. Here are some excerpts:

"…One of the most challenging and unpredictable assignments that a military officer can have is to work in partnership with a civilian. Of course, much depends on the civilian. In my experience, Mr. Tarpin was equal to ten other civilians combined. Who knew what he would do next?"

"Damon accompanied my men and me to Vietnam to kick off studies in the Ninth Infantry Division. Almost immediately, he learned the hard way about the difference between an incoming and an outgoing artillery round. Experiencing battle fatigue, DT (as one of the sergeants began calling him) decamped to Saigon, where he expressed the need for a mini R&R (rest and recuperation). I took him as my guest to the *Cercle Sportif*, the French country club… We (went) to the dressing room to change into our swimsuits. He had a giant fistful of Vietnamese currency with him, which he decided to hide in his shoe so that he wouldn't have to take it up to the pool area. After several relaxing hours and a like number of beers, we got dressed and walked back to our Jeep. It was then that DT noticed that his money was missing. He blamed the dressing room attendant whom we had spotted on the way in. Over the next few days, he complained of excruciating pain in his right great toe. He was sure he had gout. The pain became unbearable during a Jeep ride back to the Ninth

Division. So he took off his shoe to keep it from pinching the tender area. The shoe accidentally dropped from his hand. The force of the fall dislodged a wad of piasters in the exact shape of the toe of his shoe. The gout disappeared forthwith."

"The Army decided that we made a pretty good team and therefore sponsored a field study of pyoderma in Colombia, South America, in the early 1970s. Because I was military, and because we wanted to study Colombian Army units, it was necessary to brief the US Army colonel who was the military attaché at the American Embassy in Bogotá. The colonel was seated at his desk, looking somewhat skeptical, as Damon and I sat across the room on a couch behind which was an American flag. DT, perceiving the need for a sales job, began recounting his years of experience working with the military. Suddenly, I sensed that something was wrong. Looking over at Damon, I noticed that, in waving his cigarette around to make a point, a glowing ash had fallen on the flag, which started to smolder at the edge. I tried to make eye contact with him to discreetly indicate what was going on, but he was having none of it. It was then that a long ash hit the lapel of his jacket. He was utterly unaware. The hole in the flag gradually approached the size of a cannonball. It was then that the stench of burning jacket wool became apparent. DT thereupon noticed that his jacket was on fire, that the flag was on fire, and that the colonel was now taking it all in. The briefing ended abruptly. As the colonel ushered us out of his office, he promised to support our project as long as we kept quiet about how it came to be that his flag had been destroyed before his very eyes."

"As DT has said many times, anybody can have bad luck. But I, for one, have had wonderful luck with my mentor and friend who, as it turns out, has been worth any ten professors in college or medical school."

Following his retirement, Damon moved to a mountainous rural area of southeastern Ecuador where he keeps busy and his mind active while becoming extremely knowledgeable about growing flowers. I saw him there while visiting South America in 2007 and again during a special trip to Miami in 2009. The second occasion was to help celebrate his 80th birthday. Scores of his former colleagues, students, and FEST team members came to pay tribute to the man who had meant so much in their lives. The boy from the wrong side of the tracks in Southampton, England, had come a long, long way in subsequent years.

THE EVERGLADES

In a way, it started when I filled in the second—and last—dream sheet of my military career. "Dream sheet" is Army slang for a standard form for assignment preferences. The operative caveat is that at least one of the choices must be "consistent with the needs of the Army." In practice, they seldom are.

The first time around I specified England, Germany, Italy, Japan, and Hawaii—and got Vietnam. The second time I knew I was going back to Vietnam, this time with the Special Forces component of the Walter Reed Army Institute of Research, commonly referred to as the WRAIR (as in "rare"). This time there was a list of choices, a veritable smorgasbord of exotic tropical diseases like malaria, elephantiasis, cholera, dengue, rickettsiosis, sprue, and plague. The odd item in the list was skin diseases. Because of my opinion at the time of the specialty of dermatology, I placed skin diseases last in my rank-ordered list of preferences.

Over the next several weeks, my colleagues in the Global Medicine Course at the WRAIR got word of the diseases on which they would conduct research in Vietnam. I didn't. I waited and waited. Still no word, and the four-month course was coming to an end. Then, one hot and humid late July afternoon in the District of Columbia, where the WRAIR headquarters was located, the answer came.

Uncharacteristically, I had ducked into the officers' club for some air-conditioning and a cold beer before heading home. Inside, kibitzing with a bartender and a couple of fellow officers, was Major Llewellyn Legters, Medical Corps, a rare soldier-doctor, head of the WRAIR Special Forces team and therefore my new boss. As soon as he saw me enter the bar, he came over and said, "I've been meaning to contact you about your assignment. Now will do. Let's talk."

He started by saying that he had just returned from a three-day trip to the University of Miami in Florida, where he had a tour of the medical research facilities and an extremely fruitful set of discussions with one of the professors. The professor was a microbiologist in the department of dermatology. Upon hearing this, my heart sank. My face must have revealed my inner anguish because Major Legters immediately said, "You'll really like working with Damon, er, Mr. Tarpin, because of his enthusiasm and hands-on way of conducting research. You'll be going to Miami for a six-week orientation before going to Vietnam. Mr. Tarpin and his department head,

Dr. Harvey Blank, are under contract with the Army for research on disabling skin diseases among military personnel in the tropics. I have selected you for this assignment not only because I believe you'll carry out the assignment well but also for the reason that you're the only new team member to have had prior experience in Vietnam. You can hit the ground running. The Army is extremely interested in this area of research because of the heavy losses of combat manpower to skin diseases, especially among infantrymen in the wet, lowland areas of Vietnam. Good luck!"

I assured Major Legters that I would give the new assignment my best effort. What I didn't tell him was that, about a month prior, I had decided to not reflexly try to change any orders or assignments that I didn't like. This was a radical departure from my prior two years in the Army. What would be the repercussions?

August and early September in southern Florida is definitely not the tourist season. Hot, sticky, and rainy, it is unpleasant for visitors from the north but ideal as a training location for those preparing for field medical research in the tropics. With mixed emotions two Special Forces sergeants and I converged for the first time at Professor Tarpin's laboratory in Miami to begin our orientation in August 1968. Despite Major Legters' ringing endorsement of Mr. Tarpin, I half expected to meet an owlish, bespectacled, sobersided introvert with an almost nonexistent sense of humor. In other words, a person who could become passionate about miniature creatures under a microscope but not much else. I was wrong in my nagging suspicions—not a little wrong but a lot wrong.

On first meeting, Professor Tarpin seemed a little diffident, perhaps explained by his limey accent that gave away his childhood years and early adulthood in England. To me, he was reminiscent of a cross between Peter Sellers and Terry Thomas, the British comedian, complete with a wide gap between his upper front teeth. He shook hands with the strong grip of a workingman, introduced the sergeants and me to his entirely female staff of six, and said he was making final preparations for our trip to the Everglades the next day. The two sergeants and I used the lull to get to know one another.

Sergeant First Class Walden was a medical laboratory technician who decided late in his Army career to join the Special Forces. Staff Sergeant Dooley joined the paratroops as a private in 1959 but decided to become a medic when his infantry company in the 173rd Airborne Brigade was nearly wiped out in 1965 during an attack by an element of the North Vietnamese Army. Along the way he took Special Forces training. He was transferred to our team after it was discovered that his outgoing manner didn't fit well in the subdued atmosphere of the WRAIR mosquito insectary.

Our first foray into the Everglades was a foretaste of what it would be like for the next six weeks: repeated sampling of each other's skin and of the environment in the swamps to hone our skills in conducting relatively sophisticated microbiology under adverse field conditions. Professor Tarpin, who at the time was an assistant professor of dermatology, had already developed a reputation for devising ways of bringing research-laboratory-based capabilities out of the academic environment and into places where ready access to clean water, electricity, and the other accoutrements of modern life couldn't be counted on to be present.

Early on we were introduced to a fungal-culture medium that could be used to see if a rash on someone's skin was caused by a ringworm fungus, also known as a dermatophyte. It was an agar gel in a shallow plastic dish containing antibiotics that would inhibit the growth of bacteria and most fungi but not dermatophytes and a few contaminant fungi. A color-indicator system in the gel told one from the other because only ringworm fungi turned the medium red. It worked wonders in dirty, contaminated field conditions. It became known as "Dermatophyte Test Medium," DTM for short. Knowing that it had been developed by Damon Tarpin, a wag pointed out that DTM could also be thought of as Damon Tarpin Medium. Damon, as he had become known by the sergeants and me, didn't object. In short order, Sergeant Dooley began referring to Damon as "DT," and the rest of us followed suit. It was a bonding experience that boded well for us working as a team.

As the days passed, the team grew accustomed to slogging through the Everglades, collecting our samples, and refreshing ourselves at the Gator Hook Lodge, an end-of-the-road wooden shack from which could be heard—full blast from the jukebox—the twangy strains of "The Orange Blossom Special. "

> ...It's that Orange Blossom Special
> Bringin' my baby back...

The big, man-eating gators in the Everglades had long since been poached for ladies' handbags, so they were not a worry. But there were still a few natural hazards around, as I inadvertently demonstrated when I took a shortcut back to the collecting point in mid afternoon. What I initially thought were sticks in a spoke-like, radial array on a hummock were in fact water moccasins sunning themselves. I was literally almost on top of them when I discovered my error, got lucky, and streaked away before they could do me in with their venomous bites.

Despite the heat, humidity, mosquitoes, snakes, and other interferences with the comforts of civilization, the Everglades held a kind of fascination for us. As we crashed through secondary roads in DT's car, as often as not we'd see a fantasy of birdlife flying up before us, including veritable giants, such as black ibises, roseate spoonbills, and pink flamingos. I quickly became a convert to bird-watching.

One of DT's friends gave his young daughters a caged raccoon to be kept at the family property in the Everglades. I was to learn months later that the 'coon was named "Captain Masters" because of its aggressive nature.

Seemingly ever-present in the Everglades' murky, shallow waters was a candidate for one of the ugliest fish on earth. Gars, or garfish, were a holdover from the Cretaceous period 100 million years ago, and looked it. Big—up to several hundred pounds, covered with large, bony scales, and with a double row of long, needle-like teeth—they appeared more than capable of tearing any one of us to pieces. We spotted them any time we put on a face mask and swam underwater. None was aggressive, but we were never sure what might trigger an attack.

The end of the training in the Everglades was marked by a beer-bust in DT's *chickee*, an open, palm-thatched dwelling made by the Seminole Indians living in the Everglades.

It was a time to look back and to look forward. We were as ready as we'd ever be for our mission in Vietnam. And we had had a special introduction to the Everglades. We had come to realize that we were not only doing dermatologic studies, we were also carrying out ecological investigations, years before the word "ecology" became a buzzword. One of our most useful references was Mary Marple's *The Ecology of the Human Skin*.

It was time to move on. We were headed to the Mekong Delta of Vietnam.

Tacoma's Aroma

In the early 1990s, when I was a couple of months away from retiring as director of the Tacoma-Pierce County Health Department in Washington State, I ran across a *New York Times* article about Carl Hiaasen, the noted columnist and author of such piercingly satiric novels as *Skinny Dip* and *Skintight*. It captured the outrage that Hiaasen feels towards the desecration of his hometown of Miami, Florida, because of its weirdness and its mindless overdevelopment. But what really caught my eye was this quotation: "Here, (in Miami), the absurd, the bizarre, the incredible, are quickly surpassed by fact." Change the locale, and those are the exact words I would use to describe my experiences in Tacoma. Had I not lived and worked for years in Tacoma, I would not believe that an entire city and its environs could be so full of sleaze.

My first impression of Tacoma was gained when driving through it on the interstate late one hot summer afternoon in the mid-1970s. Looking west towards downtown and the Tideflats industrial area adjacent to it, I was almost blinded by the blazing sun and the bright orange-yellow of the developed area. It was like staring into the fires of hell. But that was not the only shock to the senses. You could shut your eyes to the hell fires, but you could not prevent your sense of smell from being assaulted by the stench of the large paper mill standing cheek by jowl with downtown. One of my predecessors in Tacoma told me that when he raised the paper mill emissions issue to one of his bosses, the then-mayor, he was discouraged from pursuing it when the mayor said: "That is the smell of money being made."

On arrival in 1986 I quickly ran into the sleaze and corruption: A former sheriff was being released from being in prison for corruption; a former county auditor was headed to jail for graft; and there was a pervasive sense that that was simply the way things were done. As my assistant at the Health Department used to say of his hometown, Tacoma is characterized by the ditty:

"Baseball in the sun,
Cops on the take..."

My ten years in Tacoma provided a template for what to avoid in the future.

WELCOME TO TACOMA

Landing a job against long odds in the state where I wanted to relocate after retiring from the Army engendered a sense of elation. It was short-lived. The realities of Tacoma and surrounding Pierce County saw to that.

Shortly after I knew that I was headed for Washington State, I ran into a medical school classmate who had become an authority in the field of occupational and environmental health. Jerry's response to my news was quick and negative: "You are not really going there, are you?" He was aware that Tacoma had a national reputation for pollution and had been classified as a Superfund site by the EPA. This was my first encounter with Tacoma's poor reputation.

During a preliminary trip to Tacoma, I found an article in the airline magazine that highly recommended a new guide-book, *Best Places in the Pacific Northwest*. I bought it shortly thereafter. It was excellent. The part on Tacoma, the second most populous metropolitan area in the state, was remarkably brief. Tacoma was said to have "a peculiar inward-turning quality." Was this a veiled warning?

A brief inquiry via the public library revealed that Washington State had been carved out of the Oregon Territory and had a different political history than its sister state of Oregon. From the beginning there was relative harmony between the socioeconomic classes in Oregon, whereas Washington State history was remarkably full of labor strife, especially in the built-up areas around Puget Sound. During the 1930s James Farley, FDR's postmaster general and all-around political operative, publicly used the term "the Soviet of Washington," meaning of course "the other Washington," the place on the West Coast that experienced more than its share of strikes and of organizations like the IWW and the Communist Party. Tacoma was largely a blue-collar city with a major seaport. My question was: How much of the class and political divide remained in the 1980s?

The required recent photograph for the personnel files led to a chance encounter with the grim realities of Tacoma. The photographer asked if I would like to join him for a fishing trip on the sound. We trolled back and forth in the vicinity of the Tacoma Narrows Bridge, the successor to the infamous Galloping Gertie, which collapsed and fell into the water during high winds in 1940. According to historical accounts, analysis revealed that the steady 40-knot winds set up harmonic vibrations that resulted in extreme gyrations culminating in complete collapse, fortunately with no loss of human life. But the photographer said there was more to the story. According to him, the contractor used inferior building materials, which contributed substantially to the collapse. This was Pierce County scuttlebutt. But was it true? Had the truth been covered up by the powers that be? Tacoma had a long history of graft and corruption. In fact, just as I was coming in, I found out that the sheriff and the auditor had been sentenced to prison for corrupt practices.

We caught over a dozen fish. Most were so-called dogfish, sharks a yard long. The others were black rockfish, bottom feeders about a foot in length. The head and thorax of the rockfish were covered with irregularly distributed growths, tumors of a sort. The obvious conclusion was that the tumors resulted from the toxic effluent of factories at the head of Commencement Bay. No wonder Commencement Bay was an EPA Superfund site.

While accomplishing the many little tasks required of the personnel office, I chanced to meet a nurse who had been recruited from another state by one of the major hospitals to take over an executive management function. She was poised, articulate, and self-assured, seemingly a perfect person to assume the position for which she was recruited. The encounter was brief but memorable because we were starting from similar professional backgrounds and from the same premise, that Tacoma was sincere in hiring experienced outsiders to become department heads. I didn't see her again for a year, at which time our experiences had stripped away any illusions we might have had about Tacoma. She had a haunted look in her eyes. Gone was the demeanor of the poised professional. She just wanted out.

I had been there as the new health director less than a week when I got an unexpected phone call in the evening from the head of the department's personnel section. Sean didn't sound at all like his usually ebullient self: He sounded on the verge of tears as he asked: "Have you heard about the new building?" (The foundation of a new departmental administration building had just been laid.) He said that a fire of mysterious origin had completely destroyed the foundation and that he, the project officer, would have to start from scratch. Was this an omen?

I attended my first weekly key staff meeting as an observer. Also in attendance were the three division directors—representing community health, environmental health, and administration—two assistants to the community health director, the head of the emergency medical system, and a senior nurse whose title was "planner." There was no set agenda, no time limit, and no obvious decision points, just endless, inconclusive discussion about issues that seemed to arise at random. When the planner, who didn't discuss anything about planning, said it was obvious that the discussion would last into the afternoon, I simply couldn't take it anymore and excused myself from the room.

The following week, I sat at the head of the table and told the group that I had heard enough at the previous week's staff meeting to convince me to start playing an active role. I said that each attendee had a vote, but that I as the director had ten votes. I added that, in the future, meetings would be no more than an hour in length and that there would be a printed agenda. Unsurprisingly, my statements were met with stunned silence. Subsequent weekly staff meetings changed dramatically. From then on the committee was called the Executive Committee (EXCOM in bureaucratese), raising the question: What is an executive and what is that individual's function?

A month after my arrival, the department's Finance and Accounting Section became visible in two ways: First, the incumbent head, an older woman who was facing retirement, said that the position needed a professional accountant rather than a self-taught clerk like herself; and second, that the City's finance director was giving her orders as though she were one of his employees. My response was to tell staff to begin a search for a CPA and to tell the city finance director that all orders from the city were to be cleared through me. The inappropriate bossing ceased forthwith.

It was becoming apparent that the Environmental Health Division acted in a semiautonomous manner, invoking the authority of the health officer whenever it suited its aims but without including the health officer in decision making. I decided to step in when the local newspaper reported that the residents of a housing development sited near a landfill (read: a modern version of a garbage dump) were complaining to the City about gases being emitted. They wanted some form of remediation right away. Don, the savvy, experienced, longtime head of the Public Works Department, didn't think there was a major problem.

The pressure from the public was mounting. I decided to step in and called for a press conference in which Don and I would meet with a reporter from the local newspaper. I requested that the Environmental Health Division provide me with backup material. It arrived minutes before the scheduled conference. It was technical gobbledygook, poorly written at that. It was simply useless. I made a hash of the press conference. The City backed down and gave the protesters what they wanted. It was not a good day for my credibility.

At least there were some lessons learned. There were serious communication problems within the Health Department. Therefore, I should not call for a press conference unless everything had been prepared well in advance. It seemed that a communications task force was in order, and so I tasked my assistant to assemble one.

A month later, I was sitting at my desk when a realization struck me that something was wrong. It was too quiet. There was not the usual bustle and murmur of voices outside my office. It was eerie, like the calm before a storm. I went out into the hallway where the secretaries sat. They had noticed nothing. I asked to see Rick, the environmental health director, and was told that he was away for the afternoon. But, his deputy, Gene, was available.

Shortly thereafter Gene appeared. Gene was a soft-spoken, gray-haired man with a retiring demeanor. I asked Gene if there was anything unusual going on. He denied knowing anything and didn't seem the least bit concerned.

Later in the afternoon I received a tip that I should watch the TV evening news out of Seattle. The lead story on all three networks was about a health director who had failed in his responsibilities to protect the public's health from seepage from a landfill, all in currying favor with unspecified City interests. Paul, a popular young employee in the Environmental Health Division and the son of a former state senator, read a diatribe alleging that the health director had acted against the warnings and advice of his own staff. Newspaper stories the next day were predictable: good versus evil; protectors of the environment versus polluting vested interests; and so on.

Rick and I met in my office. He seemed unusually fidgety. As we talked about the incident, the story came out. Shortly after the press conference a month earlier, his staff sent him a memorandum outlining their grievances against me and threatening open rebellion if I did not change my stance. Such a document, in my experience, was commonly referred to as an "Oh shit!" letter, and demanded immediate attention. I asked Rick if he didn't see it the same way. He acknowledged that he did, but he claimed he was too busy to inform me of its existence. "For a month?" I asked. Silence and a queasy look were all I got.

We visited the five Health Board members, one by one as the law required, and recounted the story. To no one's surprise Rick left the Health Department a few weeks later and found a job at the Washington State Health Department. I never heard from or about him again. He simply disappeared into the bureaucracy.

Living in Washington State makes you aware that there are two Vancouvers: the big one, which is the crown jewel of British Columbia, Canada, an hour's drive north of the Washington State line. The other is Vancouver, Washington, a two-hour drive on I-5 south of Tacoma on the border between Washington and Oregon. It is the county seat and has its own health department. I drove down there to attend a meeting of my peers from various local health departments. While driving around town trying to get my bearings, I noticed a metallic clanging noise coming from the right front of my car. I pulled over and did an inspection. All four wheel nuts on my right front tire mount were loosened; the nuts on the other tires were tight as they should be. Sabotage? Probably. It had to come from Tacoma because I hadn't stopped on the trip to Vancouver.

As the one-year mark at the Health Department approached, I decided to take stock of my situation. In less than a year after my arrival in Tacoma, the notorious serial killer Ted Bundy's hometown, a 13-year-old girl from the part of town where I lived was kidnapped, raped, killed, and dumped in a nearby park. This was followed by a near-insurrection by employees in the Environmental Health Division, commemorated by my being read out by an employee on all three regional TV networks. Not long thereafter I was accosted by whores on a downtown street at noon. This is not to mention such things as the apparent torching of the beginnings of a new building and the botched sabotage attempt. My military experiences stood me in good stead, especially when I got caught up in Tacoma's version of unconventional warfare. I had learned firsthand about the double meaning behind the greeting "Welcome to Tacoma."

NEIGHBORS

My new job as director of the Tacoma-Pierce County Health Department in Washington State had begun just after my retirement from the Army in El Paso, Texas. I spent the weekends after my arrival in Tacoma looking for a house to buy. Years earlier I had found that I had little use for real estate agents while house hunting, so I did it myself. The old town area of Tacoma seemed most appealing. It was the upscale part that was developed and settled by the timber barons and their ilk around the turn of the 20th century. Along the crests of the low hills were exquisite views of Puget Sound.

I saw an ad by the most upscale real estate agency. It was for a modified Tudor near the top of the hill. I toured it; it needed some superficial work, but was otherwise perfect: drop-dead views of Puget Sound, leaded glass windowpanes, hardwood floors, decorated-tile fireplace, and on and on.

There was, however, something to be considered: The house and three others in close proximity were once owned by the same family and were on a lot served by one driveway. The deed clearly stated that "my house" had an easement on the drive into perpetuity, which was long enough for me. The drive was owned by a lawyer who lived across the drive. Each of the two residences was responsible for the common-driveway maintenance on a shared basis at the call of one or the other. The exact location of the easement was spelled out in surveyor's terms. What could go wrong with that? Each owner had a vested interest in cooperation with the other owner for upkeep of the drive.

I called a real estate agent friend from the Monterey Peninsula area of California to help me with the purchase. He split the commission with the listing agent and spoke well of him.

Over the next several weeks I met my immediate neighbors. Sharing the driveway with me was a lawyer and his wife who seemed pleasant enough on first meeting. He was the owner of the driveway. On the other side of my house, and facing the street, was a young doctor who was preparing to get married and have an outdoor reception just adjacent to my property. Another house in the complex was across the neck of the driveway from my home. It was owned by a couple with two young children. The man was a lieutenant colonel in the Air Force reserve; his wife was a stay-at-home mom. All were 10 to 15 years younger than I, who was 48.

One early fall day in 1986, my lawyer neighbor approached me on the driveway and said that he intended to have it repaved in the next few weeks. Months went by with no repaving and with no further word from him about the driveway. I was in no hurry about it since the paved surface looked adequate to me. Then, six months later, I returned home from work to find that the driveway had been repaved. There was no word or warning that this was going to happen. A few days later a letter from him arrived in the mail. It contained a copy of the bill and a request that I pay half. There was no reference to the fact that a sizable portion of the driveway extended beyond the area in common as specified in the deed. Was this just a simple oversight, albeit by an attorney, or a self-serving action on his part?

Giving my neighbor the benefit of the doubt, I measured the surface area of the driveway, both the area in common and the area beyond that described in the deed. Then I computed the percentage of the total that was my easement, divided it in half, and sent him a check for the amount with a "Dear Gerry" letter of explanation. A day later I received a terse, handwritten reply letter from him, addressing me by my last name as though I were a servant, and expressing his displeasure at being expected to pay for the part of the repaving that was outside the easement.

This was from a practicing attorney?

The convenient place to park for my visitors was on the easement. Several times a year my guests would inform me that a note from my lawyer-neighbor was on their windshields, instructing them that they had parked on a private drive without his permission. There was no mention of the fact that I had a "perpetual right and easement" on the part of the drive where they had parked. This, of course, did not foster neighborly relations between him and me, so therefore we did not so much as exchange greetings when we saw one another.

I had only occasional contact with my other immediate neighbors. I noted that my doctor-neighbor had a little boy. He and his mother stopped living there when he was about three. One of my personal physicians told me that "she cleaned him out" when she left him. I never saw or heard another woman at his house during the five-year period till my departure from Tacoma.

My neighbors with the two young children appeared to be salt-of-the-earth people. They took beautiful care of their house. I was surprised one day that, during my absence on a business trip, they were evicted by the sheriff. Neighbors indicated that there was some sort of financial problem.

One weekend morning I saw an ad in the local newspaper for an estate sale that was taking place the next block over from my house. I was then interested in acquiring furnishings, so I went. The "good stuff"—antiques and such—had already been gobbled up by art lovers and antique dealers, so I poked around to see if anything desirable had been overlooked. It wasn't. But I became fascinated by the tastes of the recently deceased, whom I had never met or even heard of. He apparently was a single man who lived alone and therefore was free to decorate and furnish as he pleased. He obviously had an all-consuming cat fetish. Virtually everything had a cat *motif*, from the table lamps to the wallpaper in the bathroom, not to mention the framed pictures on the walls. They seemed to represent every part of the cat family, from African lions to docile house cats. Who would've guessed that Tacoma had housed such a creature, meaning of course the late deceased?

Five years after moving to Tacoma, I had a house guest who was looking to relocate from California and wanted a look-see at the Pacific Northwest. She parked her car—a beautiful Mercedes coupe—on the easement next to my house. This engendered a flurry of windshield notes from my lawyer-neighbor. I, as usual, told her to ignore them. She spent a week or so—enough time for my "neighbor," who drove a bright red Porsche convertible, to realize that he had been equaled, if not eclipsed, in the car desirability rankings. This set the stage for an escalation of hostilities.

A couple of weeks after my house guest had left, I had a business trip back East. I returned home to find that my "neighbor" had taken the opportunity to destroy that part of a three-foot-high hedge that ran along my property line and faced the easement. He cut exactly on the property line, presumably to make the statement that he could do anything he wished within the easement. The hedge, which had stood for years before I bought the property, now had an ugly appearance for all to see, including him. Other neighbors were shocked at what he had done. I decided that the time had come for legal action.

I consulted the lawyer I had previously arranged to represent me. Ken was a member of a leading Tacoma law firm, a former City Council member, and the recorder of my Rotary Club. He struck me as a very sound and reasonable man. On his advice, and with his representation, I initiated a lawsuit against my neighbor Gerry and his wife, Rhonda. The objective was to obtain quiet title to my property by obtaining spelled-out rules for the use of the easement.

I filed a complaint, my "neighbor" submitted a response, and the matter was heard in the Superior Court. None of the judges in Pierce County would handle the case, ostensibly because one of the parties was a local lawyer, so a judge from neighboring Kitsap County was obtained. The Kitsap judge struck me as anything but a hanging judge; rather, he seemed hyper cautious, like somebody might be if they had spent a lifetime avoiding making decisions. Interesting characteristics for a judge.

The case went to trial after months of pretrial discovery—interrogatories, depositions, and the like. In an affidavit

I submitted, I made mention that I thought my adversary had a personality disorder, which might explain his antisocial behavior.

The trial lasted almost a month. My adversary was represented by a youngish man named Lou. He called in witnesses for his client, one of whom was the real estate agent who had sold me the house through my agent. Stu, who handled high-end residential real estate in Pierce County, supported Gerry's claim that I was told, in writing, about easement restrictions at the time of sale. This came as news to me. When asked to produce a copy of the document from the file on the sale, Stu claimed that the file could not be located, a very rare event in his experience with thousands of sales over the years, or so he said. The judge didn't bat an eye at this obvious overstretch of credulity. Running through my mind was the thought that I was up against not only a neighbor with a personality disorder but also the Pierce County old-boy network. Gerry and one of his brothers were heavily involved in real estate transactions, and the family was old-line Tacoma. Stu's long-term interests were patently better served by siding with Gerry against an outsider, me.

Also called as a witness for the defense was the former owner of the house I bought. She was being counseled by her lawyer-son to avoid committing perjury, something she was apparently intent on doing as a favor to Gerry. Apparently forgotten, or at least forgiven, was the fact that Gerry had, according to another neighbor, repeatedly interfered with the use of their easement to transport their daughter. The daughter was born with a severe physical abnormality called *torticollis*, or wry neck, which made her head hang far to one side and restricted her movements. In a situation that cried out for compassion and decency, my "neighbor" purportedly made life even a bit more difficult for the afflicted girl. Yet all that was put aside when the issue was with an outsider to Tacoma.

The verdict was in my favor. How could it be otherwise when the deed granting the easement was so explicit? In the two-year period between filing and verdict, Gerry was represented by two lawyers, Lou #2 having succeeded Lou #1, who withdrew after about a year. My lawyer speculated that they weren't getting paid.

Washington State law grants a 90-day window after the verdict to file an appeal. Several days before the drop-dead date, I was talking to my lawyer, who proffered the opinion that Gerry would have appealed by then if he was going to. Besides, what was there to appeal? Nevertheless, on the very last day, an appeal was filed. And, in this litigious country where patently frivolous lawsuits are rarely deemed as such by the court system, round two of the contest began when the Appeals Court said it would review the case.

Halfway through the appeals court process, which took about a year, Gerry's second attorney withdrew to be replaced by yet another young man. The Appeals Court upheld the verdict of the Superior Court.

Once again, Gerry, this time representing himself, appealed to the Washington State Supreme Court at the last minute. By that time the third lawyer had withdrawn from the case. The evident cause was that they weren't getting paid. Meanwhile, I was receiving—and paying—considerable legal bills.

Many months after the appeal to the Supreme Court, the Court replied that it was not going to review the case and remanded it to the Superior Court for final judgment. The judgment came five years after filing suit. The title was now quiet. I could sell the house and put Tacoma behind me.

A lawyer friend, looking at the overall situation, pointed out that my neighbor's behavior was consistent with that of somebody wanting to take "adverse possession" of somebody else's property. Had I not resisted, in writing and finally by initiating a lawsuit, my adversary would be in a position to claim adverse possession by using my property—the easement—as though it were his exclusively.

There followed some icing on the cake. With the lawsuit over, I got a real estate agent whose first words of advice to me were to replace the old house-heating system with natural gas. This required that a trench be dug to run a gas line up the driveway to my house. Gerry came out to photograph the work and, in so doing, raised his camera up to my face and ignited the flash. I instinctively pushed the offending camera away from me. It dropped and broke. Gerry claimed innocence. The matter was brought to binding arbitration. The arbitrator found in my favor. Despite the supposed bindingness of the arbitration, Gerry filed suit for monetary damages. This sort of thing came under the property insurance I had on my house. Unscrupulous people treated such policies as a deep pocket to be picked, if possible. My insurance company was quite accustomed to handling such claims. Gerry was after $10,000. He eventually settled for $1,000, a petty sum in light of the time that he spent pursuing the insurance money.

Finally, I could put my house up for sale and put Tacoma behind me. The house sold quickly for twice what I had paid for it ten years earlier. Between the cost of improvements and legal fees, there was little net profit. I didn't care. My primary goal was to leave behind the social pathology and xenophobia that was Tacoma. I've never returned.

Some years after leaving Tacoma, I ran across an announcement on the Internet, dated May 2003, published by the Washington State Bar Association. In it was a listing of the lawyers who were disbarred or suspended for a year. My former neighbor, Gerry, was among those suspended. According to the announcement, the discipline was based on his conduct in several investment partnerships and corporations in the late 1980s and early 1990s, just the time that I was involved in the lawsuit against him. His partners sued him. One received a $103,000 arbitration judgment in her favor; the other, her son, was granted an award of $2.4 million. The notice went on to say, "Mr. O'Herlihy's conduct violated (the applicable law) prohibiting conduct involving dishonesty, fraud, deceit or misrepresentation."

The wheels of the gods grind exceedingly slow....

POOR RELATIVES

When I was in my late teens I ran across a thick, dog-eared paperback titled *The Rich and the Super Rich*. I don't recall getting past the first hundred of the 900-plus pages, but I got the author's main idea, as expressed in abbreviated form at the outset: "The rich are different from you and me." In their world, which is different from the world that the rest of us inhabit, the rules are altogether different. They make the rules but are not constrained by them.

An example comes from the time I accepted a weekend ride to a different state from a classmate at Princeton. I was only slightly acquainted with him, just enough to hear that he was the son of a highly placed official who had something to do with the diplomatic corps. As we crossed the New Jersey-New York State line at dusk, I could see the flashing red light behind us and noticed that the car was handily exceeding the posted speed limit. I felt intimidated by being pulled over by a state trooper; my acquaintance did not. He calmly said: "Don't be concerned; I can take care of this." When the officer examined the driver's license and other pieces of identification, he suddenly dropped his intimidating manner and became almost apologetic. It was clear that my acquaintance was no ordinary mortal. Instead of a speeding ticket and a lecture, which you and I would have gotten, he got a warm and deferential farewell from the officer.

That this is how the world works was forcibly brought back to me when I took over as director of the Tacoma-Pierce County Health Department in Washington State in 1986. I didn't have much time to think about it during the first year I was there: I was too busy dealing with such things as political attacks, attempted sabotage, and a building fire of mysterious origin, not to mention the day-to-day business of overseeing a department of over 300 employees. But after the first year had passed, it became increasingly apparent that there was one theme that dominated every part of the widely disparate functions of a large public health department: money, or rather the lack of it. Public health held the short end of the stick and had become accustomed to doing so. I decided to try to do something about it.

Wealth and poverty are, of course, relative things. As head of the department that spanned the two major entities of local government, City and County, I was privy to mutterings about the Health Department costing too much of "our" money. Compared to what? This is where things financial begin to become interesting, even for the non-financially minded.

Looking at it from an overall vantage point revealed that, at the time, 1987, Washington State health expenditures were $12 billion per year. With Pierce County accounting for an eighth of the state's population, its share would be $1.5 billion. The Tacoma-Pierce County Health Department's budget was $20 million, or between one and two percent of the County's health expenditures. Was this too much or too little?

Such comparisons and ensuing questions were not well received by the politicians in charge of the purse strings. When I asked Doug Sutherland, at the time the Tacoma mayor and chair of the local health board, if I might prepare a comparison for a presentation to the Board, I was told—in no uncertain terms—not to do so. The intended comparison was simple: Since the Health Department covered both City and County, compare its budget to that of the combined budgets for each of the City and County functions such as public works, planning, and social services. However, doing so would upset the existing order, not a good thing for a politician to have to contend with.

The existing order was clearly enunciated during Doug's visit to the Health Department. When I mentioned the subject of budget, he said matter-of-factly: "All you guys get is the crumbs off the table." The existing order was that the Health Department was the stepchild of both the City and County governments. The Department was a family member, but lowest on the pole. Doug, on behalf of the political powers that be, effectively said: "Figuratively speaking, you must realize that your proper place is in the back of the bus."

Part of the existing order was how the budget pie was sliced. In the city government of Tacoma, the heads of fire, police, and public works did the slicing, being mindful of the needs of their brethren in ancillary departments such as planning and finance. A comparable arrangement existed in the Pierce County government. Both had crumb catchers to assist in doling out the crumbs to the hybrid agencies, the Health Department and the Law Enforcement Support Agency (LESA). The latter was located deep in the bowels of the County-City Building, a characterless modern structure that replaced the razed, turn-of-the-century, classic stone county courthouse.

Fate was kind to LESA. Fed by top-of-the-news TV stories, the public perception was that the country was being engulfed in an unprecedented crime wave. Crime statistics did show a rise, but it was hardly unprecedented. In response to perception rather than reality, politicians across the country threw money at law enforcement agencies, including LESA. It was transformational. LESA rose out of the bowels of the County-City Building and got new and much nicer digs of its own. The director of LESA, heretofore a retiring man who seldom appeared at City or County staff meetings, invited the directors of the other local agencies for a visit and guided tour. It was impressive. All the latest police-sheriff communications equipment and other electronics were there. No bell or whistle was missing. It was classic politico-bureaucratic overkill.

The other stepchild agency was now in a league by itself. The Health Department remained a political football to be kicked around at the whim of politicians, news media, and community "activists." Some departmental employees, especially those in the Environmental Health Division, had no qualms about establishing personal links with council members to get support for doing pet projects. A number of these had more to do with protecting the environment— an admirable goal but not within the mission of the Health Department—than with protecting human health from the environment, such as polluted drinking water. And there were the seemingly unending complaints about the department taking an overly large portion of "my" (actually the funding agency's) grant monies for administrative overhead. Never was there a standard or accounting provided to back up claims of "too much" being taken. The employees were largely technocrats, interested only in their fiefdoms, without looking at the larger picture.

Having joined the National Association of County Health Officials early on and soon thereafter becoming a board member, I was in a position to look at local public health agencies from a national perspective. It was not an encouraging view. There was a pervasive sense of poverty, of not having enough resources to do the job. There was an expectation that this was the way things worked and would forever be. To cope, it was almost necessary to take a monk's vow of poverty, chastity, and obedience. Some of the public health physicians took the position that the lack of universal health care coverage in the US was their cross to bear, even though it was not of their making and certainly more than they could possibly influence in a meaningful way. The debacle of "HillaryCare" was yet to come.

How and why public health was viewed in the US as somehow second-class was hinted at by some personal observations. A Tacoma-based physician told me, in a doctor-patient encounter, that being a public health physician saved more lives, and thus was more important, than being in his specialty. He said this with admirably feigned sincerity. I'm reasonably certain that his annual income was multiples of mine, reflecting the value that society placed our respective functions.

At a later time, I was in New Orleans attending an American Public Health Association (APHA) meeting. The meeting itself was held in a French Quarter hotel where many of the members were staying. At the hotel next door was a convention of car salesmen and dealers. As people entered and exited each hotel, even the most casual observer would notice a striking difference between the two groups. The car people were sharply dressed and in a party mood. There was color and gaiety. By contrast, those attending the APHA meeting were solemn-faced, frumpy, and dowdy. There was a kind of gray pall over them. No fun and no hope.

In the late 1980s the AIDS epidemic was emerging from the shadows of secrecy caused by its concentration among homosexual men. The disease had just been discovered by dermatologists who noted a sudden increase in a heretofore rare malignant tumor affecting the skin. It was transmitted by two means: unprotected sex, largely homosexual, and sharing of contaminated needles by intravenous drug abusers. AIDS rapidly became a major public health concern. Fear about acquiring AIDS, then incurable and resistant to treatment, swept the country.

One day I got a phone call from Seattle letting me know that my fellow health officers from across Washington State were meeting that afternoon in the office of the Seattle-King County director of health. The reason was urgent: A staff member had just learned that an omnibus AIDS bill was scheduled to be heard three days later by a joint House-Senate committee of the state legislature. Each attendee was given a copy of the draft bill, which ran to some one hundred single-spaced typewritten pages. All the attendees, save one, dutifully started reading the densely worded document from cover to cover. The nonconforming attendee—the one from Pierce County—had a parking problem and important business in Tacoma. So I glanced through the document to get the flavor of it. It was rapidly apparent that whoever drafted it did an excellent job of laying new and multiple responsibilities on local public health agencies. However, little was said about how these agencies were to get the resources to implement the legislation. A paltry $500,000 was allocated to statewide funding. As an old political hand later said, that amount of money wouldn't make it out of Olympia, the state capital.

It took 15 minutes for me to arrive at the conclusion that now was the time to make a stand for funding. I told my fellow health directors that I had a time crunch and had to leave, but I had a question to ask before doing so. Would they support me in a concerted effort to block passage of the AIDS bill unless there was adequate funding for local health departments? To an outsider, this might seem an eminently reasonable thing to do. But public health had a long history of caving in to unreasonable demands and thereby was chronically spread too thin. The answer to my question was a unanimous "Yes." I then quickly queried my local health board members, who were all for it.

The hearing room in Olympia was new territory for me, but I was bolstered by two savvy people: Tim, the head of the state's association of local public health directors, and Jen, a staff member of my health department who drafted my remarks. Tim saw to it that I was first to comment on the draft bill, and Jen had me do such things as call the bill a "hollow document" if it should ever be enacted in its present form. The state senator who was chairing the hearings looked startled. This was united and unexpected opposition from a most unlikely source: meek health directors. As I rose from the chair in the front of the room after making my remarks, the chairman pushed his microphone to one side and growled, "You're not going to get any more money." The only thing I could think of to say was "We'll see, Senator."

Within 24 hours he had done a complete reversal. He knew he couldn't back out of saying the AIDS bill was necessary, and he couldn't deny that the proposed funding was grossly inadequate. As a result, the amount of funding was increased tenfold, to $5 million. The bill was passed and signed into law by Governor Booth Gardner, who was the Pierce County executive and chairman of the Tacoma-Pierce County Health Board before being elected to state office.

Soon the parties interested in providing AIDS prevention and services were busy trying to slice the AIDS-funding pie to their advantage. Little attention was paid to how to repeat the success in future years. To them, $5 million was a windfall of great magnitude. Seemingly unnoticed was the $95 million in state funds allocated to bail out a private business venture that went belly up. The goal of the project was to cover the downtown Seattle freeway and locate shops and other businesses there.

Months later I was at a conference of county officials and was invited by the deputy executive of my county to join him and a couple of others for a drink at the end of the workday. One of the others turned out to be the former state senator who chaired the omnibus AIDS bill hearings. On seeing me, he exclaimed: "Boy, you made me mad!" I replied that it was all deliberate, and added that I was delighted by the results and would do it again in a heartbeat if given the slightest opportunity. He just laughed. Politics as usual.

Once the AIDS funding had been absorbed into the bureaucracy of health departments in Washington State, it came to be viewed—at least in Tacoma—as just another burden to be borne. It must be said that the burden was well borne; Pierce County was recognized as having the best county-based public health program in the country—the so-called AIDS Net program. However, there seemed to be no general recognition of the power of united political action to get proper, ongoing funding. We remained stuck with the city-county agreement that the funding should be 50:50 between the two governments. If one agreed to fund, say, five million dollars and the other only four million, the overall funding fell to eight million (4 + 4 = 8) instead of nine million. It was always like that; it always went down. It was a classic no-win situation.

Insight into why people would accede to such a situation came from an unexpected quarter. The Pierce County Executive expected "his boys," including the female department heads and the half of me that was county, to attend a three-day course in Seattle titled Investment in Excellence. I was reluctant to attend, in part because it occupied the entire weekend.

The course was held in a posh setting for 400 attendees in a downtown Seattle hotel. The staff was evenly split between noticeably attractive young women and overly sincere-looking men a generation older. They were the mentors. The star of the show—and the only speaker for three entire days—was Lou Tice, the founder of an institute devoted to excellence and a former high school football coach gone inspirational.

Lou spouted pop psychology through four fifty-minute sessions on Friday morning. According to him, the "investment" was good for nearly everything, from organizational management to saving or enriching one's marriage. I felt that I'd had about enough and decided to skip days two and three. But then a funny thing happened.

The first hour of Friday afternoon was devoted to self-esteem and the effects of a lack of it. It, too, was pop psychology, but with a difference. It answered questions I'd been carrying around unanswered all my adult life. Why, for example, did a handful of professors in medical school single me out for harsh and, I believe, unwarranted treatment? Each of these episodes had something in common: I respected neither their specialty field (especially psychiatry and obstetrics) nor the professors themselves. Although I never said anything disdainful to any of them, I knew enough about myself to be aware that my facial expressions and body language were dead giveaways. But why professors should feel threatened enough by a mere medical student to use their superior positions to mete out retribution had been a mystery to me.

Lou Tice's key to unlocking the mystery was to view such situations from the standpoint of differing levels of self-esteem. According to him, people of relatively low self-esteem feel threatened by those of higher self-esteem. To make themselves feel more comfortable, those with lower self-esteem will do almost anything, including using a higher organizational position, to discredit the source of discomfort. One of my several virtues (or vices, depending on your point of view) is to have a rather high level of self-esteem and a tendency to state that the emperor has no clothes. Thus the reason that I flunked junior-year psychiatry when I did everything my fellow students did (except perhaps keeping my feelings strictly to myself). And so forth.

Tice stressed that most of this esteem-related behavior emanated from the subconscious. People were just doing what seemed natural and necessary to them. He said hardened criminals in prison routinely try to kill prisoners convicted of child molestation so as to feel better about themselves. But this did not mean that harmful esteem-related behaviors were confined to the dregs of society. It all depended on where a person's so-called comfort level was.

After the first day, I changed my mind about leaving Tice's presentations. Subsequent presentations made much of the concepts of self-esteem and comfort levels. An example was the unemployed truck driver who won millions of dollars in a state lottery. Within a year he ended up broke and in debt because he squandered the money on luxury items, expensive presents for everybody he knew, and risky investments in businesses he knew nothing about. Tice emphasized that there was nothing unusual about this situation. With less spectacular variation, it happens every day. Many people, perhaps most, just don't feel comfortable unless they're leading lives that are familiar to them, such as living in marginal

economic circumstances. Such people are eminently successful in reaching their subconscious goal—a familiar comfort
zone—even if it means living in relative poverty.

The way out, according to Tice, was to visualize success
and then to act as though it had already been achieved. The
path upward was just as full of subconscious choices as the
path down; the only difference was what the true goal happened to be.

I, for one, tried to visualize which one of the attractive
young women my appointed mentor would be. At the end of
the third day of Investment in Excellence, we assembled in
Tice's semi-mansion in Seattle, where we met our mentors.
Mine was a fortyish earnest-looking guy in an elbow-patched
tweed sport coat, not exactly what I had tried to visualize.

Whether or not I accepted all of what Tice presented
was not the point. Attendance at the course provided a new
framework with which to view public health at whatever level—local, state, or national. What I saw was not promising. At
every level I saw people willing to sit in the back of the bus.
It was almost as though they felt the crumbs off the table were
all they deserved or expected.

In their landmark book published in 1982, *In Search of
Excellence*, Tom Peters and Robert Waterman emphasized the
role of training in achieving personal and organizational goals.
This was not restricted to narrowly focused specialty training,
but was expanded to include ongoing, intensive training in
management. As befitted the predominant conception of public health departments at the time, the employees had at least
a modicum of training in their specialty area, such as public health nursing or environmental health, but little to none

in management. At my urging, the Tacoma-Pierce County Board of Health set aside monies for management training, an unusual type of expenditure. The next thing I knew, the committee of employees formed to expend the funds on management training had hired a contract outfit that provided employee sensitivity training. It was of the touchy-feely type and emphasized cultural diversity, then the new-new thing, to show one's "sensitivity" to other people. That the employees came from the most ethnically and culturally diverse county in Washington State and therefore were not breaking new ground apparently did not enter into the calculations of the committee. A significant omission was the complete absence of anything that might be considered core management considerations: budget, personnel (then recently euphemized to "human resources"), supervision, and communication.

Just as in my childhood, as a public health director I got really tired of being in the position of being a poor relative. In a way, the misfire in the management training was the last straw. I began to look forward to getting vested in the retirement system and announcing my retirement.

WHERE'S THE FIRE?

In retrospect, it seems like it was a warning shot. It happened when I was a colonel stationed at the medical center at Fort Bliss, El Paso, Texas, in the mid-1980s. When my boss—the commanding general of the medical center—had a schedule conflict, I was chosen to represent him at a dinner where the other attendees were mostly the heads of El Paso's city agencies.

During a lull in the evening's activities, the man seated to my right turned towards me and introduced himself. He happened to be El Paso's fire chief. He asked me who I was representing and then asked where I lived. I told him the street address in El Paso, whereupon he said that I lived only three blocks from the nearest fire station. He added that, in case of any emergency, to call the fire service for the most rapid response. He then asked me to look across the room at a particular man whom he said was El Paso's police chief. He said not to bother calling the police in case of need because it would take much longer for them to respond if in fact they actually did.

At the time I thought it odd that a person who headed a city agency would engage in such commentary about a colleague. Was this a personal vendetta? Was this just petty one-upmanship? Or was there something more at stake?

I had no way of knowing that a definitive answer to my questions, especially the last one, would be forthcoming in a matter of months. I had plans to retire shortly after 20 years of active duty with the Army. I had applied for the directorship of the Tacoma-Pierce County Health Department in Washington State and was accepted. Part of my new job was to supervise the handful of employees in EMS—the emergency medical service. I had had no prior experience with EMS because it is not ordinarily part of public health responsibilities. Apparently EMS had been tacked on to the Health Department several years prior to my arrival in Tacoma for reasons of political convenience. This political act was to reveal to me the realities of EMS and one of its key components: fire departments.

My principal guide through the intricacies of EMS was Pete, the local head of the service. He aggressively pursued every opportunity to introduce me to the various facets of EMS, but especially the role of fire departments. An especially memorable anecdote was his statement that it was commonplace for emergency medical technicians from both a private ambulance service and the local fire department to arrive at the scene of a road accident at the same time. When this happened, he said that a fight often ensued over which service—public (read: fire departments) or private (read: ambulance services)—would transport the patients to the hospital. At issue were jobs.

Pete's next revelation was what fire departments did for a living. This would seem to be self-evident: Firefighters fought fires, and between fires would retrieve cats that had run up trees and rescue children who fell down wells. But this was a vastly oversimplified and distorted view, according to him. As a rule, fire departments said that their mission was fire suppression, fire prevention, and emergency medical services —in that order. But if a tally were made, the great majority of calls—over 80 percent and climbing—were EMS related and had nothing to do with fire.

To further acquaint me with the EMS coordination role of the Health Department, Pete introduced me to various fire chiefs throughout the county, including the Tacoma chief, Steve. Steve was a big, soft-spoken man with a handshake that made me aware of his outsize physical strength. He cordially received us in his downtown Tacoma headquarters, where there was a built-in racquetball court. Nothing special or new was revealed by this or subsequent visits, but it was apparent that the Fire Department was not hurting for money.

About six months after my arrival in Tacoma, I joined my fellow health officers from around the state in Olympia, the state capital. The visit featured a meeting with the interim head of the state's largest and most unwieldy department, DSHS, the Department of Social and Health Services. He was a lawyer and longtime associate of Booth Gardner, the governor. He was the governor's right-hand man for such politically sensitive tasks as temporary appointments to cabinet-level vacancies. He came across as the essence of astuteness and candor. Among the several topics he covered was fire services. He was well aware that attempts to consolidate fire and other public safety departments would be met with stiff resistance. Then he said that a strong case could be made for eliminating—or at least drastically reducing—fire departments because it was simply cheaper to let buildings burn than to intervene in the traditional manner. From a statewide perspective it simply made more sense to use insurance funds to replace the structures than to foot the aggregate cost of maintaining fire departments in every locality.

Another revelation was illuminating. Why are fire departments so active in pursuits that have nothing to do with fire? Because their core business—their *raison d'être*—is disappearing from the scene. Fire codes have done more for fire prevention than anything the fire departments' relatively puny prevention programs could possibly do. A vacuum was created to be filled, if at all possible, by EMS.

In Tacoma, the competition between the publics and the privates began to mount. Attempts to reach reconciliation before the Board of Health ended when the chairman, who happened to be the Tacoma mayor, pushed the microphone away and said in a loud stage whisper: "Too much turf."

Some months later Pete told me that the Tacoma City Council was going to take up the issue of who was going to provide EMS responses for the next contract, the fire department or a private ambulance service. I attended the meeting. A city representative said that city staff had studied the issue and found that the Fire Department could provide the most cost-effective service. I had been forewarned that "city staff" was not from some uninvolved department but was composed of members of the Fire Department.

I decided to take one of the many political risks that I took while in Tacoma. I pointed out to the council that I was commenting on the issue because of my department's involvement in EMS. I said that I found it very difficult to believe that the Fire Department would be the less costly option. My remarks were met with a stony silence, except for the mayor, who made a few conciliatory remarks. The "city staff" recommendation was adopted in rubber-stamp fashion.

A year later Pete called me to say that he was having serious difficulty in meeting all the demands for certification from the various first responders, as EMTs (emergency medical technicians) were commonly referred to. He said that requests for support for an increase in staff had been rebuffed by the responder organizations. Seeing no clear-cut options, I told him to do what he had to do. A couple of days later, sharp negative reactions surfaced. The local newspaper ran a front-page story and an editorial about the unnecessary crisis caused by the Health Department. Several City Council members were unsparing in their criticisms of the Health Department's actions. It turned out that certification had been withheld in a ploy to generate an increase in staff. The ploy badly misfired. A different management approach was needed.

After several years of devoting a disproportionate amount of effort in attempting to stabilize EMS in Pierce County, I decided that devoting further attention to it was unwarranted. Pete had left for another job and was replaced by a capable assistant, Wes. I asked my own assistant, who was well attuned to the politics and caprices of his native county, to investigate finding a way to make EMS go away from the Health Department. He found a way, I didn't ask questions, and the weight of a no-win situation dropped from my shoulders.

Serendipity dictated that I had found definitive answers to the questions raised years before by my chance conversation with the El Paso fire chief. Fire chiefs and their departments behave the way they do because they want to stay in business despite a rapidly shrinking demand for fire services. So they hold aloft their carefully burnished image of heroic good guys, epitomized by the picture of a helmeted fireman on a ladder rescuing a little girl from the smoke and flames of a second-story house fire. Meanwhile such actions have almost nothing to do with what they do for a living on a day-to-day basis.

Fire departments are extremely active politically. They participate in local elections by posting yard signs favoring candidates of their choice. Their unions, said to be the single most powerful political force in Tacoma, issue coveted political endorsements.

In return for these activities, fire departments are almost invariably exempted from budget cuts. Their members receive generous salaries, early retirement, and generous (perhaps overly generous) pensions. News stories almost always give them favorable coverage, even in questionable circumstances. As an example, a front-page article in Tacoma's newspaper reported that a fire lieutenant had unnecessarily risked his life and those of others by not following prescribed procedures in a house fire. Two days later, in follow-up coverage, he was portrayed as a hero. His actions hadn't changed; the newspaper changed course 180 degrees for no apparent reason.

What is the public getting for its very generous support of "fire" departments? Good question.

A PERFECT STORM

It was just after Halloween in 1991 when I became vested in the retirement system for Health Department employees. Shortly thereafter, I asked my assistant, Dan, to set up a meeting between my two chief bosses, Joe Stortini, the county executive, and Karen Vialle, the Tacoma mayor, so I could inform them of my retirement plans. It took over a month before a meeting could be held, reflecting in part the difficulty in coordinating two separate entities of government, which have seldom been known for their rapidity of action.

It seemed like an excellent time to retire. Not only was I vested in the retirement system, but the Health Department seemed to be on an even keel and was no longer the bucking bronco that I had mounted five years previously. It looked like smooth sailing ahead.

The seven AM meeting in a nondescript, nearly empty coffee shop on Sixth Avenue, the dividing line between old and new Tacoma, was held in early December. I told Karen and Joe that I was ready and able to retire as soon as possible, but that I would be willing to stay on for up to year while they sought a new health director. Although I preferred to retire right away, I had a strong sense of noblesse oblige about being the health director, even knowing that such a concept would be utterly foreign in Pierce County.

My soon-to-be ex-bosses told me that they needed a week to inform the respective council members so they could make a joint public announcement of my retirement intentions. I agreed to wait for their signal before talking about them with other health board members and health department staff.

Two weeks came and went with no announcement. This was slow even by government standards. What was going on? The only thing that came to mind was that Joe was caught up in the aftermath of the suicide of his secret lover, a staff aide.

More time elapsed without an announcement. The Health Department's 1992 budget was passed by the Board in December. Then, in late January, storm clouds appeared on the horizon. Terri, the director of the Health Department's Administrative Services Division, and therefore the supervisor of the Finance and Accounting Section, among other entities, strode into my office with an extremely worried look on her face. She said she had just been informed by Finance that there appeared to be a hole in the budget, size as yet undetermined but potentially a large one.

It appeared that the Environmental Health Division was expanding far more than its budget allowed for. Gary, the division director, said there was no budget problem attributable to his division. Terri had advised we take our concerns to Joe, the chair of the health board, but Gary's assurances made for a divided camp. So I told Gary to double check and get back to me ASAP.

The term ASAP has a wonderfully elastic quality that has different connotations for different people. Given the circumstances, I was thinking 24 to 48 hours, not ten days. After nearly two weeks Gary appeared in my office with an expression like somebody who has been sucking on lemons. There was a good-sized hole in the budget, nearly all of which was due to over hiring in Environmental Health.

Why this? It's a painful story to tell. Months earlier I had passed along to Gary Joe's message that his constituents were pleading to speed up service in the On-site Sewage Section. (On-site sewage is a euphemism for septic systems.) The section manager decided to hire more environmental health specialists. Most new hires wanted to work in environmental health specialties other than septic systems. Somehow, possibly through the intercession of the department's HR section, the new hires were informed that they had the option of declining to work in On-site Sewage but could opt for areas more in vogue, such as water pollution. Seeing a majority of his would-be new hires siphoned off, the manager kept requisitioning more. Over a period of many months, the size of the Environmental Health Division ballooned—but slowly.

It is at this point that I'd like to insert an analogy that is used in basic management courses. It's the frog in the beaker analogy. If hot water is poured on the frog, it immediately jumps out of the beaker and saves itself. On the other hand, if water of slowly increasing temperature is poured in the beaker, the frog does not jump out until it is fatally scalded.

The Health Department provided a case study in the frog and beaker analogy. Had somebody said something months earlier, a crisis wouldn't have occurred. But nobody did.

An outsider to the bureaucracy might suggest an easy solution to the budget deficit—cut unneeded staff. This might be possible for the latest hires, but the rest had already acquired tenure. They couldn't be let go.

At Terri's recommendation we scheduled visits to the Health Board members, one by one, as the law required. The visit to Joe, the Board Chairman, was scheduled first. We arrived at Joe's office at the appointed time only to be told by a secretary that he had developed severe abdominal pains and had left for the hospital five minutes earlier. Strike one.

On visiting a second board member, a member of the county council, Terri and I were greeted with the assertion that "I already know as much as I need to know about the budget crisis." She bade us stay nonetheless because she had set aside an hour for us. The hour was filled with stories about her junkets to West Africa while a school board member. She illustrated her stories by referring to the carved wooden figures of exotic African animals, such as zebras and giraffes, that were sprinkled around her office. After an hour of such frippery, we were dismissed. Strike two.

When we visited Karen, the Tacoma mayor and Vice Chair of the Health Board that year, the tone was altogether different. She volunteered to provide some financial assistance, as long as it was matched by the County. Ball one.

While attending a monthly meeting of County Department directors, I ran into Carl, the finance director. I told him that the Health Department had devised a plan to reduce the size of the budget shortfall from $2 million—out of a budget of 22 million—down to $400,000. Would the County consider contributing half of that so as to match funds contributed by the City? The answer was a flat no; no discussion, no nothing. Strike three.

It turned out that Joe's "stomach pains" were due to a heart attack that kept him out of Health Board business for a couple of months. When he unexpectedly chaired the April Board meeting, I decided to try to arrange the briefing that had been deferred because of his illness. I had my secretary try to set up the appointment on three occasions. The calls were taken by secretaries but not returned. I was cut off from my Board chairman.

Three more months passed. I went through the motions of my job, but things were hanging fire. In early June my secretary told me she had just received notice that Karen and Joe were on the way over to the Health Department to see me. Finally, there was to be a resolution.

The meeting was cordial. They said that the time had come for me to retire, and I replied that I couldn't agree more. We briefly mentioned the difficulties of the past six months, and Joe said, "If you'd retired last year at this time, you'd have gone out a hero." Win some; lose some.

Shortly thereafter I took off for a previously scheduled vacation trip to Mexico. While I was gone my imminent departure as head of the Health Department was announced at the June Board meeting. When I got back I was a free man—free except for a couple of holdover items: accusations against me and others of several things, including sexual harassment, and a Blue Ribbon Committee report on the issues raised by the budget crisis. Those are covered in the following two essays.

ACCUSATIONS

[Introductory note: I was tempted to title this essay "The $185,000 Hustle." I hated to use such street language (after all, I am a Princeton grad), but it certainly catches the flavor of what went on under the highly charged accusation of sexual harassment. Yet, at the end of the day, I wanted to catch the eye of those who are attracted to the term "sexual harassment" and then to reveal how it can be so easily manipulated by those with an agenda. To borrow a phrase from the Tacoma newspaper, "if the shoe fits, and (I) think it does," the word *hustle* and its related word, *hustler*, are the operative terms.]

It was my first week on the job as a surgical intern at the University of California Medical Center in San Francisco. Surgical training was essentially a six-year apprenticeship, with those who were more senior passing along to those more junior the pearls of wisdom they had gained, often at some cost to themselves. My first pearl was the most memorable. The assistant resident took me aside and said that there are certain unwritten rules to follow if you're to successfully pursue your training. The first and most important rule is expressed in an old Chinese proverb: "Don't fool around with the help." Or words to that effect.

Being young and single, I was tempted more than once to disobey the rule. But I was dissuaded by the thought of having to work with a nurse who felt jilted after our relationship didn't work out. Bad karma. The way around it was to wait until the rotation on orthopedics, say, was over, then to start dating the attractive head nurse on the orthopedic ward.

This pattern of existence was broken, seemingly permanently, by my going into the Army after my second year of surgical residency. Instead of picking up where I left off after the two years of required military service, I not only decided to stay in the Army but changed specialty fields to public health. The Chinese proverb was no longer applicable because I was no longer in a similar work environment.

Two decades later I was unattached and looking for a post-Army job, preferably in a coastal area of the Pacific Northwest. It was an extremely tight job market, in part because 1986 was the year when the rest of the country discovered the Pacific Northwest, especially the Seattle-Puget Sound area. In a job-searching visit to the area, I learned that the directorship of the Tacoma-Pierce County Health Department was coming open. I visited the Department's main building, picked up a job application form, glanced around, and noticed an attractive, well-dressed woman in the personnel office where the forms were distributed. She appeared to be in her mid 30s. To my surprise, she did not wear a wedding ring.

The job offer was tendered by the Department's personnel chief on behalf of the Health Board, composed mostly of elected officials such as the mayor of Tacoma and the county executive. Sean, the personnel chief, was affable and anxious to please. It was rumored that he might leave the Department soon when a bigger municipal job came open. A parallel rumor was that Gladys, the attractive redhead I had noticed in the personnel office, would replace him if he left.

Shortly after my arrival in Tacoma, I heard that a dozen or so Health Department employees met for a TGIF happy hour at the Salmon House, a bar-restaurant closer to downtown

Tacoma than the Department. I started going as a means of getting to know—on an informal basis—at least some of the 300-plus Health Department employees. Every time I went, Gladys was already there, chatting animatedly with several others. Shortly after I sat down on the other side of the bar area from where she was sitting, she left that area, came over to the nearest seat to me, and started engaging me in conversation. It was not subtle. Although I enjoyed her company, I kept in mind the Chinese proverb.

Months passed. I settled into my new job and learned how politicized such a job could be. A well-orchestrated political attack on me was rebuffed when the attackers were outnumbered by supporters, including Gladys and her coterie. Then, on a sunny Saturday in May, in the charming little town of Steilacoom where she lived, Gladys and I found ourselves alone in a bar-restaurant after completing a march for a worthy cause. I decided to put the Chinese proverb aside and proposed that we start dating. She immediately accepted and said, "I was just about to give up (on chasing you) because I could see that it wasn't going to get me what I wanted."

We started seeing each other once or twice a week. I informed the head of the Administrative Services Division of the situation, which included the personnel contingent, in case rumors started flying. I added that I would respect the chain of supervision and not involve myself personally in Gladys' work life. I pointed out that I was unalterably opposed to nepotism.

A month after we started dating, we spent a weekend together in Vancouver, British Columbia, where we saw the house in which she had been raised and visited the spectacular farmers' market at Granville Island. On the ride back to Tacoma, she introduced me to the Joshua Tree album by U-2. Life was good. We talked about many things during the four-hour drive, including where we would go from there. I mentioned that, in my opinion, if we continued seeing each other and were becoming serious, it would be a good idea not to work in the same department. The implication was that it would be up to her to leave, as there were many more personnel positions around than health department director-ships. I mentioned that this was simply food for thought. She seemed in agreement to consider it. I thought she had prob-ably thought through the ramifications of our dating long ago.

Our next date was scheduled a week or two later at my house. It was on a Sunday afternoon. Gladys arrived attractive-ly dressed in an informal white outfit. Instead of exchanging greetings, she immediately launched into what seemed to be carefully chosen remarks. "I know you're expecting me to stay, but I'm not. Our relationship, if that's what it was, is over. Don't try to revive it. It won't work. I'm leaving now." And she did.

Her words came as a complete surprise. What was even more disturbing was the expression on her face. It was as though she had been terribly wronged and she simply wanted out of an untenable situation. She left no doubt that I was somehow the cause of her distress, but provided nothing in the way of clarification.

For the next few days, I tried to figure out what was go-ing on. I could accept that somebody wanted to break off a relationship, but I wanted to know what caused the rift. Even more important to me was what was going on behind the scenes, particularly of a political nature. I'd been thrown more than enough political curveballs since my arrival in Tacoma the year before to create perpetual wonderment if not total paranoia.

At my urging, Gladys agreed to meet me for a drink after work to discuss our situation. She seemed tense and unready to divulge what I was seeking—an explanation. She came up with an implausible and instantly forgettable reason. I met with her twice more in an attempt to hear something plausible, but it was not to be. I didn't know if my error (I assumed that it was my error) was one of commission or omission, if I did something that clearly I should not have done, or had failed to do something that I obviously should have done.

Nevertheless, several months later, I received a chatty postcard from Gladys, who was in Europe on vacation. It was sent from Paris and featured a picture of three nude young women strolling down the Champs-Elysées. It was sent to my office address. I thought it was of questionable judgment to do so and mentioned this to her when she returned. She excused herself by saying that she had no choice because she did not have my home address. This seemingly minor event was to be of greater significance years later.

Years passed. Virtually my only contact with Gladys was an occasional doubles racquetball game at noon. Sean, the personnel chief, left the Health Department for a personnel job in a small town in Pierce County. Gladys became the acting chief of the personnel contingent, now referred to as the Human Resources Section. There was talk of who would become the new permanent section head. In light of the importance of personnel specialists in interpreting the web of regulations governing a government department such as ours, the Health Department's Executive Committee unanimously recommended a nationwide search for a suitable candidate. To avoid any possibility or appearance of undue influence from inside the Health Department, the recruitment was handed to the county personnel department, and the director of that department chaired the selection committee.

Gladys let it be known that if she did not receive the appointment one way or another, she was going to sue. She ended up not being a finalist in the selection process. Another woman was chosen. The die was cast.

The proposed Health Department budget for 1992 was adopted without incident in December 1991 by the Board of Health. In late January the administrative director informed me that she had just learned of a hole in the budget. Over the next three weeks, it became clear that the hole was 1.6 million dollars in a $22 million budget and that three of the Department's 18 sections were involved, one being Human Resources.

Gladys made good on her vow to sue shortly after I had retired at the end of June 1992, five years after we had dated. The suit named the Health Department, me as the director, my assistant, the director of the Administrative Services Division and the former chief of personnel, Sean, as the defendants. Gladys was the lead plaintiff of a group of six present and former Human Resources employees, five of whom were female. The suit alleged sexual harassment. It sought an unspecified amount of damages and punitive assessments, but rumor had it they were seeking over a million dollars.

The suit was announced with some fanfare. It was the lead story in the six o'clock news on two of the three major

TV network affiliates in Seattle. The third station did not air the story, possibly because it was facing sexual harassment charges of its own from a former female employee. It was the lead front-page story in the *Morning News Tribune*, the local newspaper.

Gladys was the chief spokesperson for the plaintiffs. In the TV coverage, she claimed that the suit was a last resort because the alleged harassment, chiefly by the former personnel head, went unchecked for years. She also claimed I had retaliated against her because she had "dumped" me five years earlier. She was echoed by two other Human Resources employees, who claimed that what they had been subjected to was intolerable. It was a performance worthy of a soap opera.

The closing remark by a woman reporter on one of the TV stations was "If the alleged harassment was as bad as alleged, and had gone on for so long, why wasn't it brought to the attention of people who were in a position to do something about it?" It was a question that was never answered.

The recently retired head attorney for the City of Tacoma joined the Seattle-based law firm of Preston, Thorgrimson and served as its Tacoma representative. The firm was hired by the Health Board to represent it. Bob, the retired City attorney, thereby became the spokesperson for the defendants from the Health Department. A TV clip showed him saying that the allegations required more investigation and that the facts would come out at trial. Bob and I had a later telephone conversation in which he estimated that, as a minimum, a trial would cost $300,000 in legal fees alone and would last a month. He added that it was a clear case of legalized extortion. I didn't disagree.

Now that the case was filed, it was time for the discovery phase of the litigation. The idea was to find out what cards the other side was holding. Affidavits were passed back and forth. Depositions were scheduled. An all-business woman attorney from Preston, Thorgrimson posed the questions to Gladys and her colleagues in the presence of their attorney, who had acquired a reputation as a plaintiff's attorney in sexual harassment cases.

Depositions went on for months. Every few weeks a large package arrived from Preston, Thorgrimson containing transcripts. Gladys spent four full days being deposed. She admitted to exchanging lewd greeting cards and other sexually explicit items with fellow employees, the very kind that she and her co-plaintiffs said was one of the main bases for the lawsuit. When the depositions had been completed, it was clear to me that "see no evil, hear no evil" were the watchwords within the group. It was as pure a case of a double standard as I could imagine.

Here is a sample of what the discovery revealed:

Gladys presented Sean, her first-line supervisor, with a packet on which was written in her handwriting: *Sean, Let me warn you that this is definitely XXX rated. Don't attach my name to it please. But, enjoy—you pervert. See you when I get back. G.*

The packet contained pornographic material under a cover titled "Swedish Erotica." One page showed silhouette images of 12 nude heterosexual couples in various positions of copulation. Another showed close-up photographic images of nude heterosexual couples. One image was of a woman performing fellatio, and the other was of a man inserting his penis into the vagina of his partner, whose face was contorted with (feigned?) ecstasy or pain.

A judge and jury would not be presented the facts. We defendants were spared being deposed because the plaintiffs' attorney indicated that her side might be willing to settle, a position that she had not held prior to the plaintiffs' depositions. It was agreed between the parties to participate in mediation with a retired judge presiding.

I told Bob that I wanted to attend the mediation proceedings in order to learn what was going on in a case that involved me, among others. Bob advised strongly against doing so, saying that mediation proceedings are just short of a free-for-all and the mediator's job is to pressure those in attendance to contribute to the settlement. The last thing I wanted to be pressured into doing was to contribute even a cent to what I considered an outrage, and so I reluctantly decided not to attend.

The mediation produced a settlement. It was agreed that the Health Board would authorize the payment of $185,000 to the plaintiffs to settle the case with no admission of guilt. There was no hint in the news coverage of it possibly being a nuisance suit and settled as such.

The mediator sent an upbeat, self-congratulatory letter to the Health Board announcing the settlement. He said that both sides were to be congratulated and were satisfied with the outcome. He certainly did not speak for me.

In the fall of my retirement year, 1992, I hopped in my car and took off on a six-month cross-country odyssey. It gave me a chance to reflect on all that had happened during my six years at the Health Department. A prominent part of my reflections was being publicly accused, and then sued, over false allegations of sexual harassment and retaliation. What was wrong with our society that allowed such outrages to occur?

As I was driving along in southern Alabama on my way to the Florida Panhandle, I experienced a revelation. It was one of those instances when a person suddenly finds the answer to a longstanding, nagging problem, an answer that seems obvious in retrospect. It was a plausible explanation of why Gladys did what she did.

The explanation was as follows: Just as I had thought, Gladys had a genuine interest in me from the start, although not for the reason I thought. It was not about my pretty face; it was about my job and what I could do to further her career. She had not counted on my attitude towards nepotism. She probably had been influenced by reading then-current accounts of how the careers of attractive young women suddenly soared when they caught the attention of the CEO. Mary Cunningham at the Bendix Corporation was the prime role model in the 1980s.

With that insight, other things involving Gladys began to fall into place, especially when she first ran for state representative in 1990. News reports on the day after the election had Gladys ahead of her opponent by a narrow margin. In all probability she had been elected, but there were some write-in ballots that had not yet been counted. Gladys strode into my office the first thing in the morning, planted herself in front of my desk, leaned over on it, and tauntingly asked if I had read the morning paper. Her body language and facial expression completed the unspoken message: "You're no longer the top dog around here. I am. Get used to it." I responded by saying that I had read the newspaper and seen that not all the ballots had been counted. That election was the first humiliating loss for Gladys. The second was two years later when she ran again and lost by a wide margin. That, and repeated difficulties in finding a better job, likely stimulated her to want to counter the image of being a loser.

A fixture of my odyssey was to spend the night in motels and eat take-out meals while reading a book. My reading supply was getting low so I replenished it in a roadside bookshop. Prominently displayed was the latest page-turner by Michael Crichton: *Disclosure*. I bought a copy. The plot revolved around the protagonist, a man, getting caught up in corporate intrigue largely because of the machinations of an unscrupulous woman, a former lover. It is set in Seattle, some 30 miles up the highway from Tacoma. Two features of the story remain in my mind: The woman uses phony accusations of sexual harassment to further her agenda; and she manipulates her way out of it when the truth is finally disclosed. I felt that I had lived the story from beginning to end.

Here are excerpts from *Disclosure* that seem particularly pertinent because of the sexual harassment suit:

- "...a lawsuit will bring all this out into the open. It'll be in the papers and on the evening news for years before the trial begins. I can't adequately describe how destructive an experience that is. ...Many families don't survive the pre-trial period intact. There are divorces, suicides, illnesses. It's <u>very</u> difficult."

- "Sexual harassment had the advantage of being a charge that was difficult to recover from. You were presumed guilty until proven innocent—and it was hard to prove innocence. It tarnished any man, no matter how frivolous the accusation. (It was) the most powerful accusation she could make."

- "I hear things like, 'You can't go out with the people you work with.' Christ, if I couldn't go out with the people I worked with, I'd still be a virgin. That's all anybody can go out with—the people you work with. That's the only people you get to know."

- "...the accused has problems, too. A harassment claim is a weapon...and there are no good defenses against it. Anybody can use the weapon...and lots of people have."

Capping this off is an *Inside the (Seattle) Times* article in 1994 by the *Times* executive editor, Michael Fancher. He discusses journalistic fair play and quotes a John McCarron of the *Chicago Tribune*: "For the price of a filing fee, you can inflict serious, even irreparable harm on someone's reputation by filing a suit or administrative complaint alleging any kind of nefarious conduct. It makes no difference whether the allegation is true, because you do not have to win the case to inflict damage. The press will do it for you."

The *Times* managing editor, Alex MacLeod, was quoted as saying: "We amplify and validate these claims without even attempting to apply the journalistic standards we would if we didn't have the legal shield provided by court documents. If we're going to do that, it seems to me we have a heightened responsibility to at least follow the claims with the same enthusiasm, if not attempt to independently verify—or disprove—them."

No truer words...

THE BLUE RIBBON COMMITTEE

I can't say I wasn't warned.

It all started during a particularly contentious monthly Tacoma-Pierce County Health Board meeting in April of 1992 when I had been the Health Director for nearly six years. The source of the contention was the revelation that there was an unexpected $1.6 million hole in the Health Department's $22 million budget. This implied staff and therefore service cuts in order to close the hole. Potentially affected providers and their clients were there to express their concern. Perhaps most important, jobs, the Holy Grail of American politics, were at stake.

In the midst of this, the local head of the NAACP asked to speak to the Board. In ringing tones, he claimed that it was intolerable to consider cuts of even one dollar when lives were at stake (they weren't). He called for the formation of a Blue Ribbon Committee composed of prominent citizens from the community. The committee's function was to review the proposed service cuts and make recommendations concerning them. The Health Board immediately adopted the recommendation and called for interested citizens to volunteer their services to the committee. It seemed to be a typical political response to drain off some of the heat from a political hot potato.

At roughly the same time, the City of Tacoma, largely in the form of Karen, the mayor and alternate chair of the Health Board, commissioned a financial/management study of the Health Department by the management consultant firm of Ernst & Young. The stated point of the study was to look at management practices and financial matters to see if improvement was needed in order to use allocated monies to maximum advantage.

On the surface, both courses of action seemed reasonable under the circumstances. The Blue Ribbon Committee (BRC) would look at the specific public health services provided by the Health Department, while Ernst & Young (E & Y) would handle the financial and administrative side of things. Who could disagree?

A politically savvy person with intimate knowledge of state and local government departments in general, and the Tacoma-Pierce County Health Department (TPCHD) in particular, contacted me within days after the Health Board meeting. The message was urgent and unequivocal: Do whatever you can to stop or seriously deflect the two initiatives, especially the BRC. The given reason: They invariably engage in department bashing and underhanded methods to score political points. I replied that it would be virtually impossible for me to alter the course of events, both because I was a lame-duck director as a result of announcing my retirement and because the Health Board membership had changed substantially during the past year or two in ways that were not helpful to me as a director.

A month later I was told by my secretary that the BRC was having its initial meeting at the Health Department that afternoon. I welcomed the 18 members to the Department and pledged full cooperation with the committee as it went about its business. I was acquainted with half the members. One of my acquaintances, the union rep, mentioned to the group that it would be logical and the best use of their limited time to start with me, the department director, because I would be the only one with a complete departmental overview. I assented. Immediately afterwards, another acquaintance, the executive director of a local nonprofit called the AIDS Foundation, countered that, because of their limited time, it was doubtful that the BRC could spare the time. This non sequitur was left hanging. I recalled that a year earlier she had become hostile to the Health Department in the form of the director of the division that dealt with AIDS and me. She had asserted that her agency was more efficient at providing services than was the Health Department. She did not provide figures to support her assertion. I figured that it was another sour grapes money pitch.

Weeks went by and I was not contacted by the BRC. At weekly executive committee meetings, I asked the members— chiefly the division directors—if the BRC had contacted them. When I retired at the end of June, none had been contacted.

The E & Y financial/management report arrived the week before I retired. It was mostly prosaic but it did present information from a telephone survey of four major health departments in Washington State. In the absence of formally recognized norms and standards, analysis of the data provided de facto norms. They showed, for example, that the TPCHD was right in line with the other departments in terms of management-to-staff ratios. Nevertheless, the report continued to imply that there was too much overhead (no specific data here). If so, it is likely that the other health departments must be out of line, too. This escaped mention in the E & Y report.

The E & Y report went out of its way to inform the reader that its mandate was confined to management and finance and not to specific Health Department programs. These, the consultants said in four different parts of the 25-page report, were the province of the BRC and would be reported separately.

The E & Y consultants recommended 24 top priority administrative overhaul tasks at the same time as it called for a reduction in the staff to do them. They did not mention how this was to be accomplished. I figured that it was a sop to the "do more with less crowd" and was not to be taken seriously. Not a word was said about the specific causes of what led to the investigations in the first place—the unexpected hole in the departmental budget. The key question was, of course, whether the budget crisis was a one-time event, like a freak storm, or the first symptom of a serious underlying malady.

At the end of the summer I returned to Tacoma from my camping and fishing trip in Montana. Waiting for me was the BRC report and the local press coverage of its release. Despite the considerable misgivings I had because of the warning I'd received and because of the BRC's obvious avoidance of the Health Department's executives, I still hoped there would be something other than bashing and unsupported conclusions. After all, the committee members I was acquainted with were fellow physicians, Rotary members, and other seemingly upright citizens.

Confronting the BRC and E & Y reports was a new kind of exercise for me. I had no experience in such matters and, perhaps for this reason, I was intensely curious as to what was to come.

If the intent of the BRC was to discredit the Health Department and its director (me), then, in my opinion, it did an excellent job. The headline and the front page of the local section of the *Morning News Tribune* on September 3, 1992, read "Health Department strongly criticized." The article said "the agency suffers from a number of problems, including a lack of clear direction from the director and top management, poor management practices, excessive overhead and sup- port service costs, and poor financial practices and controls." A full-column editorial two weeks later was titled "Health Board gets sharp wake-up call." The editorial closed with "the best cure for the department is to hire a director with strong management skills and ability to command respect from the troops." With public criticism like this, I felt lucky that I had retired and was not in the job market.

One part of the editorial particularly attracted my atten- tion. It read "amid complaints of poor employee morale and mismanagement, department director Allen Masters sub- sequently chose—or was forced—to retire in June, months earlier than he had planned." Not only was this a snide re- mark, it was not factual. I had stated, publicly and in writing, that I intended to retire within the year 1992, not at the end, as the newspaper had mistakenly reported. Rumors of low mo- rale were apocryphal and just as hard to pin down. So much for the newspaper's mantra, printed on page 2A each day, "Accuracy is important to us at the *Morning News Tribune*."

Having read the words that the press had to say about me, I turned to the reports that led to the press coverage. The first was the Ernst & Young financial/management study report, which I had seen in draft form just prior to my retirement. It was mostly prosaic and hedged with numerous caveats such as remarking that a particular deficiency was common throughout local public health departments. Of particular note were several things: There were some 36 "to do" administrative items, nearly 70 percent of which were designated high priority: recommendations to cut administrative staff, the very ones whose job it would be to carry out the tasks; and the results of a telephone survey of four other major local health departments across Washington State. The point of the survey was to compare staffing ratios, the key one being the ratio of management to staff. The TPCHD ratio was 1:6, right in line with the other departments surveyed.

Having seen the press coverage, I was particularly interested in seeing how the BRC came to its strongly worded conclusions, such as excessive overhead and support service costs, and the health department not functioning at a satisfactory level in the past. Both of these conclusions had a strong "compared to what" quality. At least I thought so before I read the BRC report.

The BRC's method of arriving at its conclusions was new to me. It raised relevant questions—efficiency, duplication, cost comparisons, and so on—stated that extensive fact-finding was beyond its scope, and utilized anecdotal evidence to arrive at its conclusions. Without a caveat about the oxymoronic qualities of "anecdotal evidence," it stated that "administrative and clinic overhead costs take approximately

50 cents of every clinic dollar." It then apparently general-
ized this finding to the entire Health Department, so that the
public was presented this overhead figure as established fact.
Neither from the committee nor the newspaper was there any
mention of systematic collection, sifting, and analysis of evidence on this or any other item that the BRC included in its
purview. Nor was there any mention of a startling 50 percent
administrative and overhead rate by E & Y.

After stating that it believed significant cost savings could
be achieved by contracting out services, the BRC stated that
actual comparisons between Health Department costs and
those of other providers were not possible. I looked in vain
for why not. However, I was back to my by now old friend,
anecdotal evidence, which was alleged to suggest that other
providers can provide services at a substantially lower cost
than the Department. This nuance, a nonexistent cost comparison, was lost on the newspaper, which presented the
matter as a done deal.

The more I read the BRC report, the more I realized that I
lived in a different world from the committee. The report stated that "a wealth of knowledge about the health department
was possessed by the BRC," yet it apparently was unaware
that the Health Board and the Department had been presented the Institute of Medicine's landmark report, *The Future of
Public Health*, years earlier and was implementing its recommendations since that time. In fact, the TPCHD was the first
health department in the US to be briefed on the report by an
Institute of Medicine (IOM) representative prior to its publica-
tion date.

Under the rubric "Evaluation of Department Programs," the BRC report stated that "the committee agreed that it was not qualified to make recommendations regarding specific programs (emphasis in the original) offered by the department and did not attempt to do so." It provided no hint as to why the committee judged itself not qualified. Did not the committee consider itself possessed of a wealth of knowledge about the Health Department? Didn't the committee's membership include, among a variety of others, three doctors, a doctor's spouse, the executive director of Tacoma's AIDS Foundation, and the executive director of a social services agency, Safe Streets? Did not the BRC "have an interest in and knowledge of health department operations"?

I looked in vain for a reason why the BRC was unqualified to make specific recommendations. The only reason I could find—drawn not from the committee's report but from my own experience—was that being specific opened yourself to a barrage of accusations of being insensitive to the plight of the poor, insufficiently attuned to the needs of the community, et cetera, et cetera. I had been so successful at stirring up the wrath of clients and providers (nice people do not call them special interest groups) that I was treated to a full-bore political cartoon on the editorial page of the local newspaper featuring a white-coated health director (me) chasing away a haggard-looking mother with a waif in tow. The fact that I had not worn a white coat or used a stethoscope the entire time I had been in Tacoma didn't seem to bother the scribes and their overseers at the newspaper. Nor was there ever a scintilla of acknowledgment of the irony of editorially condemning the move of certain services out of the Health Department when the Department had recommended the moves, and later praising the idea of such moves (without specifics, of course) when they arose from the BRC.

I had originally harbored the notion that the purpose of the BRC was to provide political flak coverage for moving certain services out of the Health Department. The underpinnings of such moves were to be provided by the approach specified in the Health Board's resolution authorizing the BRC. The BRC was to "examine the efficiency and effectiveness of...services delivered by the TPCHD as related to the delivery of like services in the community...." Such a logical approach, I thought. But again, I was not on the same track as the committee. Nowhere in the BRC's 42-page report was there such a cost comparison. That did not seem to trouble anybody but me.

Both E & Y and the BRC expressed concern over duplication of effort. Obviously, this was to be deplored if it was not justified. They reported suspicions of duplication, almost always in support services. However, neither the BRC nor the local newspaper detected the elephant in the room, a situation of the BRC's own making. While decrying duplication of effort, the BRC not only duplicated the efforts of E & Y, it made a side-by-side comparison of the latter's 36 findings and recommendations. Then it did E & Y one better; it added 20 more. What was the rationale for such duplication? Why did not the BRC devote its energies to gathering the cost comparison information? Even after re-reading the BRC report numerous times, I still did not understand. It was not for nothing that I recently downloaded onto my Kindle *Alice in Wonderland*. What solace it was to read a 19th-century allegory depicting the upside-down and backwards world one encounters in stepping through the looking glass. Such was the situation I encountered in Tacoma. Clearly, I was not ready for the trip. I was not Alice.

As I drew away from the BRC report, I was struck by its reliance on the Institute of Medicine's book, *The Future of Public Health*. The committee seemed to get the message of what needed to be done, but it seemed to turn a blind eye to the difficulties of meeting all those needs. Somehow it missed or ignored the major point made in the beginning of the IOM book: "Neither among the providers nor the beneficiaries of public health programs is there a shared sense of what the citizenry should expect in the way of services." Instead, it castigated the Health Board and especially the Health Department's management. Nowhere was there context, a "compared to what" outlook. It appeared that my informant was correct: Such committees can and do use their formation as an excuse to bash the agency they supposedly are there to help.

The situation reminded me of US Supreme Court Justice Louis Brandeis' quote: "The greatest dangers to liberty lurk in the insidious encroachment by men (and women) of zeal, well-meaning but without understanding." All that was needed was for me to substitute "public health" for "liberty."

As my last act having to do with the Health Department, which I had headed for six years, I decided to write a critique concerning the aftermath of the 1992 budget crisis. It focused on the Blue Ribbon Committee report, the Ernst & Young financial/management study, and the *Morning News Tribune* press coverage. Its purpose was to provide the other side of the story, to show that the accounts that had been provided were full of holes. My motivation was twofold: one, to serve as a catharsis for me, and the other to be an educational resource for those interested in the functioning of local government and the community in times of crisis.

Just before leaving on my six-month, cross-country odyssey in mid-November of 1992, I mailed copies of the 23-page critique and a Letter to the Editor to the members of the Health Board, the executives of the Health Department, and, of course, the editor of the *Morning News Tribune*. When nothing appeared in the newspaper, I called the editor a month later to see why. He said that he had received the mailing and decided to send it to the reporter who had covered the story. He claimed to have had no response from the reporter.

As time passed, it became apparent that the mailing had met with neither a bang nor a whimper. There was just dead silence. Could it have been that the report was too sharply worded or that it brought up painful memories? Perhaps it was that the Letter to the Editor was too pungent because it contained language like the closing sentence: "Accepting this (that the Health Department is not what it was made out to be by the BRC and the MNT) will require a change from the stereotypes, attitudes, and prejudices of the past, the kind of change that seems hard to come by in this community, renowned for its odor, its crime, and its perverse politics."

Upon re-reading the critique and the Letter to the Editor 20 years after I wrote them, I felt that I had expressed myself truly and clearly. Whether Tacoma benefited from them to any degree, I may never know. But I have recently learned that the Russell Investment Company, the publisher of the widely used

Russell stock indices and the last major business in Tacoma, has left for Seattle. And Tacoma remains the crime capital of Washington State. These economic and social events indicate that Tacoma and surrounding Pierce County are losing ground, perhaps because they cling to the same shady politics and questionable practices of the BRC. Could it be pure coincidence that these events occurred while the co-chair and chief spokesperson of the BRC was a state representative from Tacoma?

I wonder.

Away From It All

Like many people, I have a tendency to be a workaholic. As the term suggests, this condition is not good for an afflicted person's health and well-being. The question is: What to do about it? Or, perhaps, what *can* be done about it?

I do not know of a one-size-fits-all answer to these questions. But I do know what has worked for me.

The first thing to do is to recognize this tendency in yourself and take it seriously. Get rid of the notion that more work will lead to a better result. It will simply lead to...more work.

I found out in college that my course grades were actually higher when I took time out for sports than when I studied all the time. But the real problem with college, as noted in the introductory essay, was that it was narrowly focused and confining, and not at all conducive to finding a suitable balance between work and play.

In the summer between my freshman and sophomore years in college, I went to Europe to visit my mother in Germany and travel around Austria, Switzerland, Italy, France, and England as well as Germany. This was a duty visit rather than something I wanted to do. As an 18-year-old in an isolated, non-coed college, seeing the sights of Europe took a backseat to dating, where I could understand the language.

Truly getting away from it all had to wait until I was 24 and planning to enter my last year of medical school. Crossing the US border into Mexico and spending two months in the most fascinating parts of the country was a tonic. I realized that, for me, near-total immersion in another country and culture was something I had to do in order to feel like I was living a worthwhile life.

Forty years later I was living in my stone cottage in southwest France as a partial expatriate. The experience of renovating the house, doing much of the work myself, was sublime. I heard about other Americans who showed interest in buying a property in France but backed out for a variety of stated reasons that boil down to indecisiveness. My question to them: If not now, when? If not here, where? My experience with having the property in France has been the realization that this has enriched my life beyond calculating. The tendency towards workaholism is gone.

MEXICO

Dr. Farber's advice to me, then a freshman medical student in San Francisco, was clear: "Do whatever it takes to take off the summer between your junior and senior years and do something that you want to do. It's the last chance you'll ever have to get this much time off for the rest of your professional life." Dr. Farber, a colleague of my father during their internal medicine residency training, was well known for his wisdom and political insightfulness. So, as time passed, I was loath to ignore his advice and go back to my summer job doing research at the University of California San Francisco medical center.

The choice of what to do during that precious summer was easy: go to Mexico. The idea of exploring Mexico was planted during a post college summer job at a cannery in Sacramento. I worked alongside two brothers from Aguas Calientes catching pears from a sorting machine (*las chingadas peras*). During noon breaks we would eat our sandwiches on the lawn under shade trees while they took turns regaling me with stories of what life was like in their home country. I vowed then and there to go to Mexico when the opportunity presented itself.

In early 1962 I began preparing for the trip that summer. I bought Margarita Madrigal's book *See It and Say It in Spanish* and learned 500 words in three days, an amazing accomplishment considering that I nearly flunked high school Latin and was the only Princeton student ever to have regressed after a semester of French. Something about motivation…

Fortuitously a new generation of travel guidebooks had just appeared in the form of Arthur Frommer's *Mexico on $5 a Day*. Its novelty lay in its intended readership, the young, footloose, and un-affluent rather than the previous generation of older tourists with their Baedekers and Fodors. It was perfect for my purposes, and proved to be reliable, up to date, and accurate.

One of my step grandmothers, a psychologist in Cincinnati, established a peace-promoting organization called the Children's International Summer Village in the post-World War II era. As a consequence, she had contacts all over the world. The membership was made up of 13-year-olds with affluent, well-connected, and open-minded parents. Because of this, I contacted her, told her of my travel plans, and asked if she could arrange for me to have dinner in a Mexican family's home. Her reply was almost a shock. Not only could I have an at-home dinner with a CISV-Mexican family, but I was welcome to stay at their house in the suburbs of Mexico City. In addition, they insisted that I send my picture so they could meet me at the airport.

Architecto Hector Gonzalez Ortega, his wife, and three boys greeted me at the airport and took me to their house in San Angel Inn, one of the oldest and most fashionable suburbs of Mexico City. All were fluent in English, well educated, widely traveled, and extremely congenial. They lived in a comfortable, modest-sized house on a pretty, tree-lined street. They had two live-in servants, one of whom was called Flaca (Skinny) to her face. The food they served was international in style with little that was distinctively Mexican. Two bright red and green talking parrots lived in the backyard.

This was not an average Mexican family. Hector was the scion of a family that could trace itself back well before the break from Maximilian in the mid-19th century, a period when an ancestor lost out to Benito Juarez to become the first president of Mexico. The ancestor had to settle for being the first chief justice of the Supreme Court. Hector gave me a privately published book concerning the power struggle: *El Golpe del Estado de Juarez* (Juarez' Coup).

Hector no longer worked as an architect. Instead, he became head of his wife's family's plumbing business, which took him periodically to inspect the portion of the business that was situated in the mountains between Mexico City and

Acapulco. He said his next trip was imminent and asked if I'd like to come along. My only hesitation was when I saw him put on a shoulder holster holding a short-barreled revolver. He shrugged when I asked him if he anticipated trouble. It was my first exposure to the realities of the Third World.

When we were about halfway to Acapulco, we turned off the main road to pick up two men, seemingly laborers, and transferred to a Jeep before starting up a mountain on a private road. We encountered several closed gates; when we did, the two men jumped out to open them. Higher and higher up the mountain we went, through thick vegetation interspersed with the blooms of wild orchids. Finally we reached a clearing where there were a dozen or so primitive wooden houses, each with a crudely hewn wooden cross over the front door. There were poorly dressed women and children about. Pigs and chickens wandered in and out of the dwellings. We had reached the settlement whose men were the labor that supplied the wood for the toilet seats sold by the plumbing company.

We spent the night in a whitewashed communal building on mats covered by a blanket. We ate and conversed by candlelight. One of the outside men who joined us pointedly asked me to guess how old the older of the two laborers was. I replied that he looked about 35 to 40, but was probably younger than he looked because of the effects of a laborer's lot in life. With a grin, the outside man, probably one of Hector's relatives, told me to ask Juan his age. Juan said he was 86 and could remember being a soldier at the turn of the century. Only then did I notice that there was a fleck or two of gray in his hair and a slight stiffness in his hips when he walked. Was I witnessing a virtual miracle, a hoax, or just an unusual situation that provided entertainment for a few men on a mountain? I will never know.

The next day Hector and I drove down the mountain, exchanged the Jeep for the car, and headed for Acapulco. Hector said that his family had been going there for vacation since 1927, a time when travel was by horse-drawn carriage. After getting a hotel room, Hector insisted that we visit the first high-rise building in Acapulco, which housed the *Club de Pesca* (Fishing Club), the most prestigious social organization in town. Instead of taking me in for a drink, Hector toured me around the outside of the building and went on and on about the architectural design and building details. I didn't suspect that I was being set up. When we'd completely encircled the building, Hector asked me to look at the ground in front of us. There, on a cornerstone engraved in bold letters, was the name of the architect, Hector Gonzales Ortega.

After two days of seeing the highlights of Acapulco, including the dives off La Quebrada cliff over a hundred feet above a surging sea, Hector returned to Mexico City and left me to fend for myself. A couple of days later, while waiting for a bus, a hard rain started falling that forced me and more than a dozen other Americans my age into a nearby bar for shelter. We planned to leave for the bus as soon as the rain stopped. We had to wait for hours. So we socialized, broken only by repeat drink orders and frequent trips to the toilet, necessitated because we all had the *turista*.

As we got acquainted, one of the young women in the group attracted the attention of the men because she had an irresistible aura of sexuality about her. She was not particularly physically attractive—her orange dress did not flatter her, and she was not the least bit coquettish; nevertheless, she had an effect on the men as though she were pouring out pheromones by the bucketful. As a result, one member of the group, a Yalie who wanted you to know that he was an Eli and therefore entitled to the best in life, couldn't stay away from her. This didn't make any difference until the rain stopped in the early evening and the bus took us downtown. Unbeknownst to the Yalie, Ms. Orange Dress had a date that night with the owner of the most chic restaurant in Acapulco. When Ms. O D entered the restaurant, the Eli was in hot pursuit behind her, and apparently oblivious of the two burly men in tuxedos standing near the door. Even the most casual observer would notice a bulge near the left armpit of each man. When Ms. O D was greeted by her date of the night, the Yalie didn't take the hint, even when the two tuxes suggested that he do so. The last any of us ever saw of him, he was being "escorted" out of the restaurant, the soles of his shoes two inches above the ground.

A few more days of the Acapulco scene made me long for something more traditionally Mexican, so I got a bus ride to Taxco, the city known for its silver, just west of Mexico City. While there, I was invited to visit the home of a young saleswoman in a silver shop. For Mexico, it was probably middle-class housing; in the US, it would be rated a slum dwelling. Another introduction to the Third World.

Soon I found myself back in Mexico City at the house of my new friends, in part to attend to practical things such as laundry, and in part to see the attractions in the area around the city. Just down the road from San Angel Inn was the

university, whose building walls were covered with the flam-
boyant murals of Diego Rivera. Just east was the fashionable
suburb of Coyoacán, where I saw the former house of Leon
Trotsky, a politically prominent Russian exile, who had a falling out with Stalin and was assassinated in Mexico in 1940.
Further east was the city of Puebla with its 365 churches, one
for every day of the year. Hector said to pay special attention
to the decorations on the walls and ceilings of the interiors.
The craftsmen were Indians who had recently converted from
their tribal religions to Catholicism. The results of their efforts
was a mixture of two almost antithetical religious traditions;
the down-to-earth symbolism of the Indians, for whom ears of
corn meant fertility, contrasted with the Spaniards' use of the
cross as an ineffable expression of their spiritual aspirations.
Clearly the religious and cultural conversion was incomplete.
I got the impression that no attempt to understand Mexico can
safely ignore this fact.

Hector told me that he had recently contacted his cousin,
the chief of tourism of Chiapas, the southernmost state, which
borders on Guatemala. He said that I should visit Chiapas,
make contact with his cousin, and things would proceed from
there. Indeed they did. I soon found myself in the remote
mountain town of San Cristobal de las Casas at the home of
Frans and Trudy Blom, a Danish-Swiss couple who had emi-
grated to Mexico decades earlier because of their interest
in the culture of rural Mexicans, especially the remnants of
Mayan tribes who inhabited the untamed areas of Chiapas.

Upon entering the large living room, I saw a man who
looked like he was from a different world. It turned out he
was. He was a Mayan chief whose band lived in the jungle

surrounding the mountains. He had been flown out with his 15-year-old daughter-in-law, who had sustained a gunshot wound to the jaw. He sat on the edge of a chair, obviously very ill at ease in his surroundings. He muttered Mayan words, spat on the floor when it suited him, and darted his eyes around the room. He was dressed in a dirty white smock, and his thick, straight black hair hung down his shoulders and back. Upon noticing my reaction to seeing the chief, Trudy said that he was much more savage when he came out of the jungle two weeks earlier; considerable effort was required to train him where to go when he had the urge to urinate and defecate.

Trudy quickly found out that I was a medical student. She said the doctor hadn't come back to see the wounded Mayan girl since his initial visit two weeks before, and that the wound was oozing. As the only medically trained person around, would I please come see the girl? I agreed, of course, and didn't think it would be fruitful if I tried to explain that I had only finished my third year at an academically oriented medical school, and that consequently I had next to no experience in managing a patient with a serious wound.

Night had fallen when we entered the tiny, ultra-primitive 400-year-old hospital. Light was furnished by candles. A middle-aged woman referred to as an *enfermera* (nurse) was hovering about. It was obvious that she was not a nurse in the modern sense of the word, but more of a barely educated and trained practical nurse. The patient was lying on a cot, with a dirty white chunk of cloth taped to her lower jaw and a fearful look in her eyes. I was in completely over my head. The only thing I had to offer was a show of caring. I took the stethoscope proffered by the nurse, despite the rubber tubing being three times too long, and appeared to listen to her chest. I couldn't hear a thing. Even if she had had roaring pneumonia I wouldn't know given the various limitations at hand. After a few minutes of this charade, I tried to assume my most professional demeanor, and said that I thought it urgent that the doctor come to see the patient the first thing in the morning. The eventual outcome? I've always wondered.

At the urging of Hector's cousin, I arranged to fly to a recently uncovered Mayan temple site deep in the Chiapas jungle. Tourist facilities were in the early stages of development, but there was a small "hotel" where one could find bed and board. As I approached it I saw a small child outside who squatted down and, in the absence of any clothes but a shirt, had a large and extremely liquid bowel movement. I immediately became more concerned about developing a massive case of *turista* than studying the intricacies of a Mayan temple. It turned out that there was ample time to study the temple because it took four days of waiting for my turn to fly back to civilization.

With my appetite whetted for remnants of ancient Indian civilizations, I continued my travels by bus and visited Monte Alban and Mitla near Oaxaca; Chichen Itza and Uxmal on the Yucatan peninsula; and the giant stone heads of the Olmecs south of Veracruz. It drove home the point that the Aztecs were simply the latest in a series of Mexican Indian civilizations that dated back thousands of years. While brutal as combatants, they were anything but savage when it came to architecture, astronomy, mathematics, pottery making, irrigation agriculture, and calendrical dating and recording of historical events.

Everyday events were often revelatory of Mexican culture. One day I decided to walk to my next destination, thinking it was only a couple of kilometers away. To make sure, I asked a young woman on the side of the road if the next town was very far. *"O, no, señor, no esta lejos. Esta muy cerca."* (No sir, it's not far. It's very near.) So instead of looking for a bus or a taxi, I walked...and walked...and walked...until I found the town over ten kilometers away. I then realized that I had made the mistake of not asking for the distance, but for an answer that would be pleasing (It's nearby) or not (It's far away). This woman's culture was part Spanish, and courtesy, especially in dealing with strangers, demands the pleasing response.

Another time I went shopping in a large, covered marketplace. I was dogged by a man who wanted to sell me some tourist trinkets. I kept saying no, I didn't want any. He kept pestering me. Finally, in a fit of pique, I said to him, *"Chinga tu puta madre!"* (translation not provided, but the expression had something to do with his mother). This was simply to get his attention and thereby get rid of him. But it was heard and relayed by people nearby, and a hush fell on the entire market. The trinket salesman looked enraged. The people around were giving me hostile glances. I decided to beat a hasty retreat.

All too soon, it seemed, the summer was coming to an end. I hated the thought of leaving Mexico. I wanted to stay another year, become fluent in Spanish, soak myself in the culture. An extremely long-shot plan hatched in my mind: play the Mexican national lottery and, if I won, let the medical school know that I'd be a year late in returning for my senior year. Alas, the gods were not on my side, and soon

I was seen off at the Mexico City airport by Hector and his family. It was as close as I've ever come to feeling homesick.

As the plane flew into Los Angeles, I began to realize why I had a knot in my stomach. I was returning to blatant materialism, hyper cleanliness, glitz, a machine-dominated society, chrome everything. Gone were the reminders that life can be lived at a different pace, that there are values other than the mindless accumulation of stuff.

Thirty years later, in 1992, I revisited Mexico to see if I could recapture what it was that made it seem so attractive. The short answer is that I couldn't. I had undoubtedly changed a great deal in the intervening period, but so had Mexico. The population had doubled; *supermercados,* formerly nonexistent, were everywhere; plastic had replaced wood; American tourism was rampant; and there was a palpable loss of the distinctiveness of Mexican life. The materialistic culture of the country to the north was seeping into even the remotest parts of Mexico. I haven't returned.

ROOKIE GRINGO

Norm was a fellow surgical intern at the medical center in San Francisco in the mid-1960s. We worked seven-day weeks and grew accustomed to four hours of sleep a night. Social and personal life was practically nonexistent. The only letup during the year was the ten-day vacation.

Although it was tempting to stay home and catch up on sleep during that period, it was even more enticing to spend the time as far away as possible from the work environment. I opted to go to Mexico, a country where I'd spent the entire summer two years previously. Norm expressed interest in accompanying me. He reminded me that his only foreign travel experiences were day jaunts across the Soo into Canada from Detroit, his hometown.

We decided to go to the upper west coast, and over to La Paz near the tip of Baja if time permitted. It was spring, the plane fares were reasonable, and we were able to get vacation time simultaneously.

After checking into our hotel just before dark, we went out to explore the town. It was garishly lit and full of Southern Californians. A beachfront bar and restaurant attracted us, in part because we saw a number of fellow Americans enjoying themselves in it and also because it seemed to be the cleanest place in town. Soon we were downing margaritas and ordering food a la carte. Norm seemed to be enjoying himself immensely. Despite the pittance we were paid, he went ahead and splurged on a seafood cocktail.

Two days later we were in a hotel room in Los Mochis, a couple of hours down the coast from Guaymas, when Norm suddenly became violently ill. He had terrible abdominal cramps followed by near-continuous vomiting and diarrhea. He couldn't keep anything down. He was getting weaker and weaker.

As weak as he was from loss of fluid, he was still able to think clearly. He correctly read my mind. He knew that I was concerned about him becoming dangerously dehydrated. He also knew that I was thinking about getting him to a medical facility where he could be administered a salt solution in his veins. He remembered the horror stories we'd all heard about grossly substandard conditions in Mexican hospitals, usually expressed in such terms as "Do anything else you want, but don't take me to Guadalajara General." In a barely audible voice, Norm said almost the same thing—just the hospital had changed. Now it was Los Mochis General.

Over the next three hours, I kept checking him for the cardinal sign of far advanced dehydration—collapse of the neck veins. It didn't happen, no doubt in part because we were basically in good physical condition despite being overworked and underpaid.

Norm survived the night and was on his way to recovery by morning. At dinner the next night, he was extraordinarily careful about what he ordered. Everything had to have been thoroughly cooked. Gone was the desire for any more seafood cocktails. He had noted that I hadn't ordered any, and I hadn't gotten ill. He intimated that because of my prior experience with Mexico, I knew which foods were safe and which were not. Therefore I should have warned him about the seafood cocktail. I didn't have the wherewithal to tell him that was all a matter of price; I would probably have been as sick as he was if I was a little less frugal that night in Guaymas.

For the next several days, Norm berated himself for ordering the seafood cocktail. He said that he suspected all along that it might be risky but that he let down his guard because he was on vacation. He had no way to know about the risks right around the corner.

We found ourselves in a small town off the beaten tourist track one afternoon and decided to have a beer in a nearby cantina. The bar was empty except for a table of four men 20 feet from our table. We ordered bottles of Dos Equis. The four men were looking in our direction and making whispered remarks to one another. Suddenly one of them—fortyish, short, obese, and sloppily dressed in a khaki uniform—addressed us in a loud, mocking tone of voice. He said he was the local police chief and wanted to know what we were doing in his town. It was obvious to me that he wanted to have a little fun at our expense.

Norm didn't know any Spanish and was forced to rely on body language and facial expressions to grasp what was happening. To him, the four men appeared to be hostile, belligerent, and fully prepared to do what they wanted to do with us, however sadistic. He was as apprehensive as I'd ever seen him. He looked like he would dart out the door if only he knew where to run.

I sensed that to show weakness would only embolden the four men. So I replied to the fat lieutenant using the same bantering tone that he'd used on me. I was careful not to appear to be overly cocky, just savvy enough to know that this was a game to while away the time in a boring little town.

The ploy worked. Fatty and his three subordinates became civil and even a bit cordial. I was careful to avoid saying anything that would make the lieutenant lose face in front of his men. The Spanish I learned two years earlier was invaluable, as were the experiences I had that summer in Mexico.

We exchanged smiles and pleasantries with the four men as we left the cantina. Norm confided in me that he was filled with trepidation when he saw me stand up to Fatty and his henchmen. He thought we were goners. I replied that I wouldn't and couldn't have done what I did unless I'd spent a summer in Mexico.

Norm began to see himself as the survivor of two life-threatening events, each a variant of being at the wrong place at the wrong time. To him, our trip seemed more like an ordeal than a vacation. Could it get any worse?

We had three more days until our return flight to San Francisco. It seemed to me that we had two choices in how we would spend the time: stay safely holed up in our current hotel room or fly over to La Paz for some deep-sea fishing. I mentioned this to Norm. His gaze softened when I mentioned the hotel option, and hardened on hearing of deliberately exposing ourselves to a possible misadventure at sea. You could just read his mind: With two strikes against us, why risk the possibility of a third? He had a point.

Norm reluctantly agreed to go along with my preference that we go fishing in La Paz.

The waters of the Gulf of California, between mainland Mexico and the Baja Peninsula, had a worldwide reputation for their abundance of game fish. With any luck we would catch at least a few. The day after our arrival in La Paz, we went out on a chartered vessel with other fishermen aboard.

One of the group had a major strike. It was Norm. He hooked a large sailfish that fought him every inch of the way when he tried to reel it in. At times, it came out of the water, danced on its tail, and dazzled us with the iridescent colors of its body and the size of its sail. After an hour of alternately stripping line off the reel and then being hauled back towards the boat, the giant fish was gaffed and brought on board. Norm was exhausted from the effort of playing the fish; his arms were shaking from the strain. But it all had been worthwhile. His luck had begun to change.

When we got back to land, we found out what happened to the catch. It was hung up by its tail for photographs. Its body had lost its color and turned black. It was not valued as a food fish. There was a gnawing feeling inside us. We regretted the fate of the magnificent creature. We felt the need to turn to a different kind of fishing.

The next day we went out in an outboard with a skipper and a couple of poles. When we got to the fishing grounds, the skipper baited the hooks, then let out the line and handed a pole to each of us. Within minutes, Norm got a strike and reeled in his catch, a ten-pound fish with an extremely well-developed chest area. The skipper said they were good eating. He re-baited the hook, let out some line, and handed the pole back to Norm. Fifteen minutes later Norm caught a second fish, and 20 minutes after that, a third. I hadn't had a bite. I was beginning to develop a profound sense of paranoia.

It occurred to me that there might be more than luck at play here. Perhaps there was an unsuspected difference between the two poles in terms of the length of line let out, the way the hook was baited, which side of the boat it was on, et cetera. The way to find out was to switch poles and sides of the boat where we were sitting. Norm graciously consented to the switch, then proceeded to catch seven more of the large-breasted fish. I never got a bite. Conspiracy theories started floating in my head.

Once back ashore we arranged to give the fish to an orphanage nearby. That act effectively ended our vacation—the rest was mere processing: packing, getting to the airport, and flying. We were homeward bound, back to 18-hour workdays in an antiseptic hospital environment. Memories of our vacation jaunt to Mexico would soon fade, or so we thought.

Now, a half century later, Norm has long since become a world traveler, both on foreign vacations and as a consultant to medical centers in foreign countries. Nothing in his subsequent travels would come close to the trip to Mexico for sheer emotional involvement. Time hasn't dimmed his memories of a violent case of the *turista*, being at the mercy of hostile small-town cops, and enjoying a fisherman's paradise. He fully realizes that, at the end of ten incomparable days in Mexico, he was no longer the same person. He was no longer a rookie gringo.

MICHELANGELO IN SANTA CRUZ

Once in a great while a needle appears at the top of a haystack. It does so in defiance of the law of physics that says this should not happen, the law that gives rise to the expression "as difficult as finding a needle in a haystack." I found the figurative needle after four years of a heretofore arduous but fruitless search for it.

"It" was the opportunity to learn how to work with stone, specifically to become a stone sculptor. My yearning to become a worker in stone had been building for years, possibly resulting from periodic vacation trips to Europe where I admired the stonework in Italy, France, and Great Britain.

I started my search in Tacoma, Washington, where, in 1992, I had just retired as the director of the Health Department. I now had the time to devote to learning about stone. But where to start? Tacoma was not promising because it was a largely blue-collar, heavily industrialized port city, hardly the Florence of America. By a fortunate turn of events, I found myself staying for two months in Portland, Oregon, as part of a six-month cross-country odyssey. There, I found several well-stocked art supply shops that carried specialized books on stone sculpture as well as carving tools. It was a start, but there were no leads on where to learn about using the tools.

The most valuable thing I picked up in Portland was the dictum that, to become a visual artist in any medium, it was first necessary to know how to draw. Like most people, I not only didn't know how to draw but believed it was an innate skill, perhaps genetically dependent. In other words, if you weren't born with the knack, forget it. That this was a fallacious belief was the main theme of a remarkable book, *Drawing on the Right Side of the Brain*, by Betty Edwards, a gifted art teacher. Through reading the book and performing the graduated drawing exercises, I not only became a competent beginner at drawing but also learned how to "see" like an artist. As a typical left-brained American, I was unaware that the right half of my brain had gone largely unused as a result of my cultural conditioning. It was a momentous, almost eerie feeling to experience a shift from one side of the brain to the other as a result of following Edwards' instructions.

Two years later, in 1995, I was called back to California because of illness in the family. I decided to live on the Monterey Peninsula, a place I knew well because I had been stationed at Fort Ord in the 1970s. I joined the local arts scene—took drawing lessons in Carmel, became a docent at the Monterey Museum of Art, and looked for stone sculptors. The one I was able to find said he had just retired from teaching and did not want to take on any more students under any circumstances.

A final dead end?

Serendipity had been a fixture of my life. I sorely needed it now. It came in a most unexpected form: a monthly TV guide. I subscribed to a PBS station in San Jose in the heart of Silicon Valley. I habitually circled in ink the listings that looked promising. In the spring of 1996 I spotted a small box ad in the middle of the guide. I would never have noticed it unless I was circling something nearby. It was four summer offerings from the University of California at Santa Cruz's extension. One of the four courses was stone sculpture. My luck had changed. Or had it?

I noticed that it was a two-week course in midsummer. I had already signed up and paid for a community-college-sponsored tour of Peru. The tour did not end until the weekend between the two weeks of the sculpture course. I was not about to miss the one-time Peru tour with an exceptional guide. Seeing the Incan stone buildings at Machu Picchu was too important.

Deciding that half a loaf was better than none, I called the sculpture instructor, explained my predicament, and told him of my willingness to compromise. He said it was best if I drove up to his studio in Santa Cruz so that we could discuss it further.

It took an hour to drive from my apartment in the seaside Victorian town of Pacific Grove, following the arc of Monterey Bay to the outskirts of Santa Cruz. The Michelangelo Studio was located in a century-old former tannery. The studio's name derived from the owner, Angelo, and a former partner, Michael.

Angelo was in his early fifties, a few years younger than me. His speech marked him as a streetwise import from North Jersey or New York City. He was stocky, ebullient, and a complete extrovert with an Italian twist. Within moments after our first meeting, he said: "You do not want to take the course. Use the money you would have spent on tuition to rent studio space from me." It was a completely unexpected offer, but it made perfect sense to me. We made a brief tour of the building; he pointed out the corner space I would be using, and sent me off with a plastic bag of wet clay from which to mold a human torso to use as a model for carving a stone likeness.

I returned a week later with a rent check and a busty female torso in clay. Angelo said it would do and told me to accompany him out back where the blocks of stone were kept. He said I could choose any kind of stone I wanted as long as it was alabaster. I picked a red variety. It weighed over 200 pounds. Angelo used a hydraulic lifting device to take the stone into the space I had just rented and put it on a heavy-duty sculpture table. Because I had brought the tools I had bought in Portland, I was ready to start carving. But how?

There are some things that cannot be taught from a book, and stone carving is one of them. It requires a tactile sense that is not intuitive. Angelo quickly taught me the basics: Hold the point tool just so with your left hand; with the right hand, hold the two-pound hammer (heavier than it sounds) and strike the end of the point tool just so. Control is vital. Hold the point far down on the shank; hold the hammer down near the head, not at the other end of the handle. The angle at which the point meets the surface is crucial. Too great an angle, such as a 90-degree angle, and the stone won't be so much carved as shattered; too small an angle and the tool will simply skip along the surface of the stone. It's a classic example of the adage: Not too much and not too little, but just right.

Just as I began, Angelo disappeared. I had seldom felt so on my own. I gingerly took a few swipes at the edge of the stone block. It came as almost a surprise that I could carve something as hard as a stone.

My hand-eye coordination left something to be desired. The back of my left thumb suffered when the hammer hit my thumb rather than the end of the point tool. The answer was to develop better coordination and to start wearing heavy leather work gloves.

I drove up to Santa Cruz twice a week to work in my studio space. After a couple of months, my piece began to take shape. I asked Angelo to come by and give me some tips. Two sessions later he came by, nodded at the piece as though to say progress was satisfactory, and asked what I was going to do with my next piece. I thought I had misheard. My next piece? I was still struggling with my first one. Angelo assured me I had not misheard, then asked if I knew the meaning of the artistic term *controposto*. I replied, "That's when the human body is twisted around," and he said, "Yes, it means literally 'around the post.'" Maybe his newest student was not so retarded after all. He said, "It is a good thing you know what it means because that's what you are going to be creating in your second piece."

Angelo had a deft touch when it came to teaching. He did not hover or control; he made a quick evaluation, provided succinct advice, and disappeared. When I sensed I had reached a point where I did not know how to continue, he seemed to know it intuitively. He appeared out of nowhere, checked to see if his intuition was correct, gave a succinct suggestion, and disappeared again. It always worked.

In the ensuing couple of years at the Michelangelo Studio, I carved figures from alabaster, marble, and soapstone. My favorites were a two-foot-high Carrara marble nude figure of Eve stepping out of the Garden of Eden, a life-size marble image of my right hand holding the world, and a one-third-life-size likeness in alabaster of a mute swan with feathers arching over its back.

My sessions at the Michelangelo Studio were severed when I moved to the East Bay of San Francisco in 1999. By that time I could work independently and did so at studios where I rented space. My favorite piece from this period was an alabaster likeness of a medieval cloister capital. Instead of depicting a Bible story, as would be done to aid the monks in their religious contemplations as they walked around the cloister, I used a secular story that is part of the folklore from the area in France where I live half the year. I am reminded of it each time that I am on my back terrace in France and see in the distance a 600-foot-high limestone cliff that is central to the story. The French government has designated the cliff as a cultural attraction called the *Saut de la Mounine* (Monkey's Leap). For those who are interested, a version of the story follows this vignette.

Looking back at the two-and-a-half-year period at the Michelangelo Studio, I can see that it was one of the most transformative episodes of my life. It nourished the creative spark that heretofore was buried deep inside me. I will always be grateful.

The following story was taken from the Internet.

We (the foreign visitors) continued up a moderately long hill to the "Saut de la Mounine." Mounine seems to be in Occitan for monkey. Thus "Leap of the monkey." The story is, some local noble was upset about the company his daughter was keeping, and decided to have her thrown off a cliff by some of his servants. A local cleric, horrified (for some strange reason) by this idea, dressed up a monkey (this isn't the only local monkey story, and where they found monkeys in France in the middle ages, I'm not sure) as a young woman, and had the servants throw the monkey off the cliff instead. Seeing this from a distance, the nobleman was horrified at what he'd done, and grief-stricken for his daughter. When the cleric confessed his ploy, the nobleman was greatly relieved, forgave his daughter, and everyone lived happily ever after (apparently it wasn't an issue whether the daughter forgave her father, and the disposition of the suitor isn't discussed in the account we read).

EXPATRIATISM

The airline magazine article was titled "Tourists vs. Travelers." Instead of the usual fluff extolling the features of places that the airline serviced, the piece was remarkably insightful about how people could be divided up according to their reactions to traveling.

Tourists, according to the writer, went to their temporary destinations, shopped and took pictures, and gladly returned home with souvenirs, gifts, and of course the photos. Particularly avid tourists didn't simply visit a place, they *did* it, as in "We did Paris in the afternoon, then flew to London for dinner and a play at the Old Vic, and were at Heathrow at ten the next morning."

Travelers, on the other hand, may be seen at the same places frequented by tourists, but they experience them quite differently. They wouldn't dream of *doing* a place; they try to immerse themselves in it, to get the feel of its language, culture, and landscapes. They don't like to feel that they're on a schedule, and they're not in a hurry to go home. Theirs is a much more contemplative journey, incompatible with the snapshot qualities of postcards and slide shows.

I knew immediately which side of the divide I was on. I was a traveler and had been one since the age of seven when I took a train trip alone from St. Louis to Cincinnati. Like any member of a minority group, I sometimes felt out of the mainstream through no fault of my own. I'm the kind who would turn down a prize consisting of "an all-expense-paid trip for two to the resort at Waikiki" because I don't like beachfront high-rises, hordes of tourists, and forced fun. I don't play golf either. I am the first to realize that there is something vaguely un-American about these qualities. A traveler would understand without being told that this has nothing to do with patriotism but is a matter of temperament and personality.

It is commonplace that traveling may be part of a job, which it certainly was when I joined the Army as a two-year "obligated volunteer" and stayed in for a 20-year career in the Medical Corps. In that time, as part of my duties, I had temporary assignments to many parts of the world, including northern Alaska in the winter and Saudi Arabia in the summer. With 30 days of paid vacation a year, there was ample time and money to visit such countries as France and Italy, not to mention Turkey and Egypt.

This pattern continued after my retirement from the Army in 1986, and lasted until the year 1998. Then something happened. For the first time in my life, I no longer felt like I wanted to be a traveler. I forced myself to go on a planned trip to Ireland, which was unexpectedly enjoyable, but it was a swan song. The fire for traveling had gone out.

Just as nature abhors a vacuum, so there was a feeling of emptiness that urgently needed to be filled. And it was.

It struck me that the energy I had previously poured into my travels could be redirected to something potentially even more fulfilling. That something would, through the alchemy of the mind, turn out to be becoming an expatriate.

The very word "expatriate" has an evocative quality. To me, it conjures up images of Ernest Hemingway and Gertrude Stein in Paris, James Joyce in Trieste, and Peter Mayle in Provence. What heady company. But could I be like them, at least in becoming an expat, if not a famous person?

My mental journey towards becoming an expatriate was helped along by recalling what Stein had said about her hometown of Oakland, California: "There is no there there." Born and raised in the Cincinnati, Ohio, area, I understood her quip completely.

There were only two countries that came to mind when I considered the all-important question of where to go when I expatriated myself: Italy and France. This was largely based on two considerations: food and my love of stone buildings. Based on previous travels, I assumed that I would end up choosing Italy. Serendipity helped me along in the form of a use-it-or-lose-it round-trip ticket from San Francisco to Rome. I decided to use it to spend a couple of days in each of six

Tuscan and Umbrian hill towns that I had previously visited. I found each as charming as before, but I couldn't see myself living in any of the six for months and years at a time. Italy was out.

Serendipity, which has ruled much of my life, came along again the following year, the millennial year of 2000. It took the form of an invitation to spend two weeks in June in southwest France at the second home of an acquaintance from California. Veronica had bought the place two years previously and renovated it with the help of a bilingual English estate agent. It was a captivating place along the Lot River, complete with a tobacco hangar that had been converted to guest rooms. Centuries-old houses made of native limestone from the surrounding cliffs were all around. To me, it was a paradise. I had found the area in which I'd like to settle.

Unlike a full-blooded expat, I didn't want to reject my home country for the sake of another. Nor did I want to have a token presence, such as a vacation home, in another country. I wanted to have the best of both. The answer was to spend half my time in France and half in the US. It happens that the spring and fall are my preferred seasons in France (neither too hot nor too cold), while winter and summer in coastal California are kept at moderate temperatures because of the ocean. It also happens that France requires a visa for stays over three months at a time, and the French tax authorities may deem you a permanent resident for annual stays of more than six months. Best to stay inside these limits.

Three months later I returned for a look-see. Nigel, the British estate agent, spent a day touring me around, at the end of which I saw the house of my choice, a real fixer-upper.

The price in francs was less than US$30,000, including closing costs. Nigel said that it would take triple that to restore it. Coming from California, buying a fully restored, century-old stone house in a beautiful location for around $100,000 was unthinkably inexpensive. I decided to make an offer. It was my first major step to becoming an expatriate.

The following week I was in the office of a *notaire*, a type of lawyer who specializes in real estate. My offer had been accepted; the seller and I were there to sign the papers. Despite having taken three years of French in high school and college, I couldn't read a word of the documents. Nigel told me to initial and date each page where it said *"lu et reçu."* Little did I know that it meant "read and received." It was a wake-up call that I needed to learn French—and fast. I felt as though I had a gun to my head. Learn…or else.

Because the house I bought was more than a century old, as indicated by the date, 1883, incised in the keystone of the barn, it was necessary to get official approval of architectural plans for a remodel. Despite a couple of re-dos, the plans never seemed to incorporate the recommendations made by Nigel and me. It turned out that the head of the firm never provided them to his subordinates, and they were afraid to ask. It took months to get past this hurdle. There was a rigid hierarchy even though this was a small private business and not a governmental bureaucracy.

Finally we got plans that incorporated our recommendations. Now to submit them for approval, a process that by law could take up to 90 days. On the 89th day they came back disapproved for minor reasons. Back they went to the architect. The process was repeated. It finally ended—with approval—a year and a half after it began. Nigel said that it was always like that, no matter how many times you'd been through it. There were apparently no incentives or pressures to streamline the process, whether from the private or the public sector.

Nigel warned me that it was hard to find somebody to do the renovation because there was so much demand and so little supply. Builders were reluctant to add employees because of the extremely high upfront costs for social insurance. And it was next to impossible to let go an employee who didn't work out for whatever reason. These government-imposed mandates were made in spite of professed concern over unemployment, which of course was only exacerbated by them.

Nigel was able to find a mason to do the work. He was English and was hired not because he was a Brit like Nigel but because he was available. Keith pitched in, starting with the attached barn, which was in ruins. I happened to be visiting in April 2003. Keith volunteered that it would only take six weeks—barring additions to the scope of work—to complete the renovation. I was elated. Things were on a roll.

I returned to the US and got periodic progress reports from Nigel. The usual message was that Keith was making slow progress because he often didn't show up for work. He had taken on other jobs. I was told he had taken on the practices of his French colleagues.

I returned in the fall. Keith showed up one day and did a full day's work. Things seemed to be back on track. At the end of the day, he said: "I'll see you tomorrow." He didn't show up again for a month. I was being initiated into the realities of being an expatriate.

One of the approaches to combating this reality was to do as much as possible of the work myself. Although I intensely dislike the stickiness of paint, I did all the painting and varnishing. I made and hung shutters, installed all the lighting, and did myriad other things. Outside, I used the leftover stone from the house renovation to repair and extend the stone wall. With even more stone remaining, I made a sunken terrace and a raised garden bed. I worked 14-hour days, seven-day weeks, for months. It was exhausting but, at the same time, exhilarating.

Such projects required frequent visits to the hardware and home-improvement stores in the area. I didn't have time to be embarrassed by my French; I had to learn it on the fly. The pressure to learn helped tremendously. I now have a barn full of tools, all of which I can now name as well as use. Not a bad result.

When entering a store or supermarket, here called an *hypermarché,* a customer is almost invariably hit by a blast of sound, most of it popular American songs in English. English words appear frequently on packaged consumer items such as home electronics. As compared to American exposure to the French language, the French are almost immersed in English, much of it spoken or spelled in the American way. There is great pressure to improve one's ability to converse in English, probably stemming from the fact that English is now the universal language, the lingua franca, as it were.

It took me awhile to realize that a French person's desire to speak to me in English was often motivated not so much to increase my comfort level but by the speaker's desire to practice speaking English. Unless the speakers were clearly fluent in English, I learned always to reply in French, often with the result that they reverted to speaking in French. Turnabout was fair play.

The need to furnish my newly acquired home, as well as the need to acquire tools for repairs and renovations, provided a glimpse of how different is Europe from North America. An electric kitchen utensil or a power tool might come with a thick owner's manual, but by the time the thickness was split into 20 languages, little of substance remained. What was left more than vied with American manuals for unevenness and incomprehensibility.

Five years after signing the purchase documents in the *notaire's* office, the renovation was nearly complete. The only thing remaining to be done was to put a cover above the chimney to prevent rain from going down it and rusting my Norwegian woodstove. Keith had cemented a short stack of bricks at each of the four corners of the chimney, but, despite repeated entreaties, he never returned to put a cover on them. It became clear that if anything were to be done, I'd have to do it myself.

The limestone slab that Keith had left as a cover was far too thick and heavy to do the job. So I bought some cement and rebar, added some small stones, and put the mix in a wooden frame to cure. The weather was so cold that the concrete wouldn't set when it was in the barn. So I moved operations into the warmth of the house. I used plastic sheeting to protect the wooden floor of the dining area. Unbeknownst to me, there was a hole in the plastic, and the water from the concrete mixture leaked onto the floor. The large clear spot where the chemicals ate through the finish can be seen to this day. But the reinforced-concrete cover set perfectly.

It was one thing to have a suitable cover, and quite another thing to put it in place. It weighed well over 100 pounds, and it needed to be raised 25 feet above the ground. One man with a tall ladder couldn't hack it. Something more was needed.

Once again serendipity came to the rescue. An electrical contractor was changing the streetlight fixtures in our hamlet, a process that required a hydraulic lift on the bed of a truck. The contractor was happy to loan his lift and his right-hand man to help me place the cover on the chimney. When I asked him how much I owed him for his services, he gingerly asked if 25 euros would be too much. I gave him 40. It was worth it to cap off years of unrelenting effort to achieve a final result.

It was a fitting time to look back over the five years since I had started on the path to becoming an expatriate. Somewhere along the way I had successfully crossed the divide between being a traveler and being an expatriate. Having a fully renovated and furnished stone house in a beautiful part of southwest France was part of it. Another part was feeling as comfortable living in France as in California. Both were home.

⤳⤳⤳

Things I wouldn't have known unless I were an expatriate:

France won the Second World War, at least in the European Theater, almost single-handedly. This feat is hailed each May in political speeches throughout the land. Contributions to the victory from other nations, such as the United States, were so inconsequential as to be unworthy of mention.

It is an unwritten but nevertheless rigorously observed rule that a French person at the wheel of a vehicle must drive at maximum speed when in their home *département* but dawdle and act confused if driving in other *départements*. This rule is temporarily suspended when nearing a radar speed detector.

It is never too early to teach children how to comport themselves in a political demonstration (*manif*) or strike (*grève*). In recognition of this fact, the French primary school system encourages children as young as first graders to participate in marches while holding banners that say: Don't trample on the rights of kids. (In impeccable French, of course.)

The merry month of May in France is merrier than in any other country because there are three official holidays, all scheduled for Thursday. Any *artisan* (craftsman) worth his salt always takes the following Friday off so that he has a four-day weekend. Anybody who avers that s/he will get a building project completed or plumbing leak fixed during May is promptly institutionalized for insanity.

Airing of grievances and labor strikes are national pastimes in France, especially by members of unions that can cripple an industry or service, such as the SNCF, the French national railroad. The train line from Toulouse to the town nearest my home is critical to going to and from my homes in France and the US. When the first SNCF strike interfered with my travel plans, I hoped that the ensuing bargaining session would resolve the problem for years to come. By the third strike in the same year, I began to get the picture: This was no unusual streak of occurrences; this was a way of life.

Americans are programmed to look at trips outside the country as short visits for either business or pleasure.

Explaining that you are leaving for a three-month stint for the purpose of working seven-day weeks to restore your home in France is invariably followed by the cheery sendoff: Have a nice vacation.

PECH-MERLE

I live half the year in Southwest France. The most prominent feature of the landscape is an array of vertical limestone cliffs that rise from the river valleys. Some, like those seen from my back terrace, soar 600 feet above a bend in the River Lot, which flows westward from its source in the *Massif central* (central mountains). The limestone derives from countless numbers of calcified endo- and exoskeletons of creatures that lived in warm, shallow seas during the Jurassic period, some 175 million years ago. Subsequent movements of the earth's crust elevated the seafloor to its present levels. The rivers cut through the limestone to form canyon walls.

At times the river meanders close to the base of a cliff. This constricts the width of the country roads that parallel the river. Early on, I was driving along such a road and saw three young men dressed in what seemed like wetsuits walking on the other side of the road next to the cliff. Suddenly they disappeared. As I passed the place of their disappearance, I saw a large crevice in the rock just above and parallel to the surface of the ground. The conclusion was obvious. The men were spelunkers and the crevice was an entrance to caves hidden in the limestone hills. This was my introduction to the word *karst*, which is the German word for a limestone plateau where erosion has created underground caves and streams. The erosion is caused by eons of slightly acidified rainwater percolating through fissures in the rock. The acid comes from rotting vegetation at the surface of the plateau.

I found out that there was a karstic cave complex just a 45-minute drive west from my house. It was Pech-Merle (Blackbird Hill) near the small town of Cabrerets along the River Célé, a tributary of the Lot. It and its larger cousin an hour away to the northwest, Lascaux, are world famous for their cave paintings. The chief difference between the two is that, while there are more paintings in Lascaux, visitors are not allowed to see the originals because of breath-related damage to the paintings. In contrast, visitors can take escorted tours at Pech-Merle and go to the small but well-curated museum on the grounds.

Pech-Merle was discovered accidentally nearly a century ago by two local boys and their dog. They entered through a preexisting access point. Their chief problem was in combating the ink-black gloom of the cave's interior with only a torch. Now visitors enter through a recently created edifice complete with a stairway to descend into the cave. There are electric lights throughout the cave complex, which stretches nearly a mile in length.

For first-time visitors the experience is literally almost unimaginable. There, on damp limestone walls, are dozens of paintings, some created 25,000 years ago and all completed by 10,000 years ago. The artists used ground charcoal for black pigment and iron-laden deposits for a rust color. They mixed the pigments with their saliva and sprayed it on by mouth to create silhouettes of their hands. Other techniques, such as mixing pigments with tallow or using a stick to apply paint in a more controlled fashion, came later.

The world that the artists depicted was far different from the world we know today. The world they knew was of ice sheets and tundra with fauna to match. With the exception of scattered indecipherable symbols and a few stick figures of humans, all of the depictions are of large mammals: There is no flora, no action taking place, and no ground to stand on. The animals are invariably shown from a side view. And they are gloriously rendered. There is no difficulty in identifying bison and bears, for example.

It is helpful to remember that the people who created the cave art were hunter-gatherers whose very lives depended upon having an intimate knowledge of the animals they depicted. The large animals were their prey. As mythologists such as the late Joseph Campbell have pointed out, there was a close relationship between the hunters and the animals they hunted. There was much more to it than simply having meat to eat.

A dozen large mammal species are depicted. Of that number, almost half became extinct by the end of the latest ice age 10,000 years ago. No longer are there hairy rhinoceroses, cave bears, and mammoths, for example. They died out in a geological minute. Among paleontologists there is a heated ongoing argument as to what caused the sudden extinction. One camp blames climate change, the opposite camp says it was due to overkill by human hunters, and the in-betweens say it was due to a bit of both. There is evidence both ways.

Not all of the depicted animals went extinct. The horses and cattle are still with us, although in altered (e.g., smaller) form in the case of cattle. Reindeer are now pretty much confined to the Arctic Circle, where the tundra is conducive to their mode of existence.

The depictions of humans, few as they are, are startlingly different from those of animals. There is no attempt to portray their actual appearance; there are only stick figures. They almost always show men in armed conflict. The most memorable is of a man who has put a spear through the torso of another. It is impossible to decipher the emotions and motivations of the combatants.

While visiting Pech-Merle it becomes apparent that the term "caveman" is a misnomer. Because it is always cold (50 degrees F), dark, and damp in the cave complex, it would be impossible to dwell in. One would go only to visit, and then only to create an inviolable sanctuary to safeguard the most treasured and respected of the representations of their culture. It is at heart a religious experience and so impossible to convey its full meaning to someone who is from an entirely different culture and of a vastly different time.

The museum is an important adjunct to the cave. The 20-minute film is well done; it shows the early days of the cave's discovery and offers interpretations of the paintings. Since the cave paintings were created by Stone Age people, it has a display of stone tools, beginning with the earliest and therefore crudest types to the highly refined tools that evolved just prior to the Age of Bronze. As one who has tried his hand at fashioning stone tools such as arrowheads and axes, I can vouch for the amount of labor and degree of skill required to create a usable tool.

A visit to Pech-Merle is a reminder of how much the material world has changed in the 25,000 years since the first paintings were made at that site. It also shows that the underlying themes of human existence have changed not at all.

Climate change, warfare, and species extinction are still very
much with us. Perhaps the speaker in the Book of Ecclesiastes
said it best when he declared that there is nothing new under
the sun. However, he could have added that there is just endless variation on the basic themes.

Time and Chance

What is the purpose of a memoir? I have found from first-hand experience that this is a recurring and sometimes vexing question in the mind of the writer. In compiling this memoir, I think I have found an answer to the question.

For me, the purpose of writing a memoir is to probe one's memory in such a way as to allow the most forceful memories to make themselves felt, to push them to the center of one's consciousness. Then they can be recorded and examined. It was not by accident that I started this memoir with my recollections of brushes with death. These were the most forceful and vivid memories I had.

Both during and after composing the first-person essays that constitute this memoir, I kept wondering: What is the meaning of these episodes in my life? What can others learn from them? Is there an overarching message?

The key word here is wisdom, as in the wisdom of Solomon, the biblical king of the Hebrews a millennium before Christ. Solomon is thought to be the author of the biblical Book of Ecclesiastes, which deals with the meaning of life. According to the writer, who described himself as Teacher,

"All is vanity."

As the memoir neared completion, I kept thinking of Ecclesiastes. I had to agree with Tom Wolfe, the author of the best-selling novel *Bonfire of the Vanities,* when he said: "Ecclesiastes is the greatest single piece of writing I have ever known, and the wisdom expressed in it is the most lasting and profound."

Long before I ever read Ecclesiastes, my life experiences had convinced me of the truths contained therein, above all the following lines:

> The race is not to the swift,
>
> Nor the battle to the strong,
>
> Nor bread to the wise,
>
> Nor riches to men of understanding,
>
> Nor favor to men of skill:
>
> But time and chance happen to them all.

CPSIA information can be obtained at www.ICGtesting.com
Printed in the USA
LVOW06s1018270713

344940LV00001B/1/P